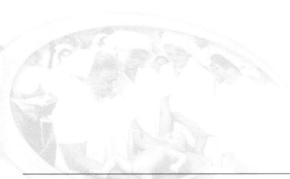

ON REVOLUTIONS
AND REVOLUTIONARIES:
25 YEARS OF REFORM AND INNOVATION
IN NURSING EDUCATION

Pamela M. Ironside
PhD, RN, FAAN
Editor

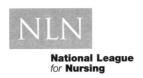

National League
for **Nursing**

National League for Nursing
61 Broadway
New York, NY 10006
212-363-5555 or 800-669-1656
www.nln.org

ISBN 9781934758397

Cover design by Brian Vigorita
Director of Marketing Communications, Laerdal Medical Corporation

Printed in the United States of America

ON REVOLUTIONS
AND REVOLUTIONARIES:

25 Years of Reform and Innovation in Nursing Education

Dedicated to the Revolutionaries:
a small group of passionate teachers who pooled
their individual efforts to reform nursing education,
their wisdom, dedication and foresight to create a
national movement

And to all Revolutionaries present and future:
who bravely leave the comforts of tradition and work
tirelessly with students and colleagues toward excellence
by transforming nursing education and practice

TABLE OF CONTENTS

The publication of this volume would not have been possible without the support, encouragement, and contributions of many. The editor and contributors wish to acknowledge the following:

The National League for Nursing – an organization that has demonstrated unwavering support for nursing faculty, excellence in nursing education and nursing education research directed toward preparing the nursing workforce to meet the needs of diverse populations in an ever-changing health care environment. The willingness of this organization to critique its positions, programs and processes made the original Curriculum Revolution possible and paved the way for the transformation of nursing education now and into the future.

The contributors, past and present, who gave so generously of their time to create a dialogue between the original Curriculum Revolution and the contemporary context of nursing education.

Elaine Tagliareni and Terry Valiga for their vision and persistence in making the idea of this volume a reality and for their unwavering encouragement of all faculty to challenge assumptions and transform nursing education.

Em Olivia Bevis – a consummate educator who was known for her intellectual prowess, vision, and sense of humor. She is greatly missed.

Lisa White, Sandi Fowler, Ben Johnson, Brian Vigorita, and Karen Klestick for their technical assistance and support throughout this process.

Joanne Ashley – a master teacher who gave nursing a resounding wake-up call to bring feminism to the very center of our consciousness.

On Revolutions and Revolutionaries:
25 Years of Reform and Innovation
in Nursing Education

Introduction

Pamela M. Ironside and Theresa M. Valiga

Nurse educators across the country are facing significant challenges borne of critical shortages of faculty (particularly those with preparation as educators), diminishing resources, increasing diversity in student populations and program options, competition for clinical practice sites, and persistent growth of both nursing knowledge and technologies infusing education and practice. Concomitantly, there is growing concern among health professions disciplines and the public about the safety of patients seeking health care services, thus increasing scrutiny of the readiness of new nursing graduates for contemporary practice. These concerns are reflected across institutions of higher education, where calls for more faculty accountability for student progress and learning outcomes are becoming commonplace. These are certainly extraordinary times, and the persistence of these challenges harkens a renewed interest in substantively reforming nursing education.

Calls for reform and innovation are not new in nursing education, and the National League for Nursing (NLN) has historically been at the forefront of reform efforts. In 1973, the NLN launched the Open Curriculum Project (Notter & Robey, 1974; 1975a; 1975b; 1976, 1979) as a way to mobilize nursing educators to initiate reform to improve their schools. This initiative focused on having schools demonstrate their ability to accommodate the diverse learning needs and career goals of students by providing flexible opportunities for entry into and exit from the program. The project resulted in the development of advanced placement testing, the acceptance of more open (flexible) admission and progression procedures, the design of innovative curricular models, the evaluation of various approaches to achieving an open curriculum, and the dissemination of study findings (Notter & Robey, 1979).

In the following years (1988-1991), the NLN launched another major reform initiative entitled the Curriculum Revolution. This undertaking provided opportunities for teacher-scholars to engage in shared dialogue about the future of nursing education, to seriously question the pervasive reliance on outcomes and competency-based models in nursing education, and to advocate for substantive and sustained innovation in schools of nursing. Presentations at the four Curriculum Revolution conferences and the subsequent research and scholarship highlighted how the underlying assumptions of *any* approach to teaching and learning influence the content, instructional strategies, and evaluation methods selected by teachers. Awareness among faculty grew as leaders highlighted and critiqued the unintended consequences of these choices in the preparation of nurses in general and the experiences of teachers and students in schools of nursing specifically. Leaders argued that substantive reform would not occur by merely switching, swapping, or sliding content around (see Chapter 4) or by rearranging the deck chairs of content on the Titanic of nursing education (see Chapter 8). Rather, an examination and critique of the underlying assumptions of conventional and alternative pedagogies in nursing was necessary.

The Curriculum Revolution served as an impetus for teachers across the country to initiate and extend reform in their curricula, in teacher-student relationships, and in the community within and outside the school of nursing. It also fostered attention on how new pedagogies based on phenomenology, critical social theory, and feminism could enhance nursing education. Indeed, we now have new pedagogies for nursing developed from nursing research (Diekelmann, 2001) and a growing research base documenting the contributions of diverse pedagogies in nursing education (Falk-Rafael, Chinn, Anderson, Laschinger, & Rubotzky, 2004; Ironside, 2006).

It is easy in hindsight to view the Curriculum Revolution as a moment in time or a short-lived trend in the history of nursing education. One might consider it to be merely a series of conferences where leaders in the field provided guidance and direction for those seeking to reform their courses and schools through implementing the latest innovation. It also is easy to make judgments about the successes or failures of this historical era through the lens of "what we know now" and the tangible or measurable difference this collective work made (or failed to make) in particular schools of nursing or to the discipline overall. But do these views tell the whole story of what transpired and its meaning and significance for nursing education? What can one learn from revisiting initiatives such as the Curriculum Revolution?

The Beginnings

The Curriculum Revolution began with a group of faculty who saw shortcomings in the current approaches to teaching nursing and sought ways to substantively improve nursing education. These teachers were working in diverse settings around the country and found each other through participating in the Open Curriculum Project, networking at conferences, and by word of mouth. As these individuals planned ways to invite broader conversation about their ideas and concerns, they selected the term "revolution" as a harbinger that the focus of these events would be on *substantive* changes in curriculum design and implementation. In other words, the Curriculum Revolution was the collective expression of what was already occurring in many schools of nursing and the collective effort to create a substantive change on a national scale – a more responsive and relevant nursing education! Reflecting on this period, one of the revolutionaries recently commented:

> We didn t know what we were doing, not really, but we weren t afraid of taking the
> risk. We didn t think we were starting anything big, we just knew there had to be

a better way [to prepare students]. It s like we all shared a sense of the problems, and yet, it was a lonely time with each of us working away on these issues in our own schools with precious few opportunities to talk with other teachers about how it could be different. Frustration was high at the inertia in nursing education which really seemed to be going nowhere and the same problems came up over and over again. To be quite honest, I was ready to give up. But instead we decided to have a conference [laughs], pretty bold, wasn t it? At the time, this was just a way for me to get together with other teachers I knew around the country who I knew were working as hard as I was to find a different way. I always found it so energizing to connect with other teachers who shared a common vision, who were willing to put their heads together and talk about their thinking. And that s what it was. We wanted a place to think together and to challenge our current practices and to explore how nursing education could be different. It was like starting a journey without being particularly clear on where you are headed! But again, maybe the entire journey is in the first step.

The Revolution came to life as more than 400 faculty gathered at the first conference to dialogue and debate teaching issues, to challenge assumptions, and to envision new pedagogies for nursing. It was fueled by a belief in the collective wisdom of teachers and in the new possibilities they could create and enact by working and thinking together. It was, perhaps, a revolution in how we, as nursing faculty, thought about teaching and the implications of our work as teachers in the lives of students, clients, and communities. The Revolution *created a place for thinking together about teaching and learning and imagining a better future*. Three more conferences and four publications followed, spurring a great deal of research and scholarship in nursing education, the development of substantively new nursing pedagogies, and calls for the advancement of a science of nursing education.

The Curriculum Revolution Revisited

The contemporary context of nursing education is one in which the demands of teaching using predominantly conventional pedagogy (the most time-consuming pedagogy) frequently conflict with time for thinking. Indeed, it often is the case that teachers decry "there is no time for thinking!" The volume presented here is a compilation of essays focused on creating, once again, a place for thinking among teachers about everything present and absent in our current approaches to teaching and in proposed alternatives.

Six essays, written by several leaders in the original Curriculum Revolution, have been reprinted in this volume. Each of these essays contains a wealth of ideas and insights, many of which continue to resonate with nursing educators today. This collection of essays also gives us a glimpse of the revolutionaries' thinking and how they were struggling to get beyond tradition by creating new pedagogies for nursing education. Reflecting on these essays provides us with new insights about the risks these teachers took in so boldly calling for substantive change in a national forum and enacting change locally. Even though 20 years have passed since the first Curriculum Revolution conference, the essays included here will sound remarkably familiar – many of the issues discussed continue to be both relevant and perplexing. This familiarity will, no doubt, raise questions about the extent to which we, as nursing educators, have been successful in addressing particular issues or solving pedagogical problems.

It is clearly important for us to persistently and critically examine our past and present efforts to reform nursing education and the extent to which these efforts have been successful. It is equally important for us to concomitantly consider the extent to which such issues or problems are "solvable" in the usual sense. For example, as knowledge proliferates, teachers are faced with too much content (Ironside, 2004), making the selection of content for particular courses and throughout the curriculum appear to be a persistent problem. But perhaps content selection is not a problem per se but *is an integral part of all pedagogies*. Thought of in this way, the issue is not one of finding a "solution" to too much content, but rather one of raising questions such as: How do teachers and students think about what content to keep in a course and what to leave out? What role does memorizing content play in preparing students for practice?

What matters, perhaps, is not what content teachers select but *how it is selected*. Perhaps such issues continue to show up in our thinking and in our literature because they are not matters that can solved, but rather are matters that require our best thinking over time as we listen and respond to the evolving contexts in which students learn and nurses practice. Indeed, perhaps looking for a "solution" inadvertently curtails thinking and the substantive dialogue and debate about the relationship between content knowledge and nursing practice and how students can best be introduced to the knowledge and practice of the discipline.

Interspersed with the original essays are responses and reflections that bring these historical pieces into conversation with contemporary thinkers. These reflective pieces were graciously contributed by both original revolutionaries and by a new generation of leaders in nursing education. This conversation, created across time, is one of circling – listening back and forward through our experiences, traditions, and practices and through our concerns and questions. It is an opportunity to listen anew for how the collective wisdom of teachers can be preserved and extended in these chaotic times toward a preferred future for nursing education and a robust science of nursing education.

Keeping Reform and Innovation Alive

Since the Curriculum Revolution, there have been dramatic changes in the healthcare system and in how nurses practice. Has reform in our nursing programs kept pace, or are we inadvertently preparing students for a healthcare system that no longer exists? The need for substantive reform and the continued development of research-based pedagogies has, perhaps, never been greater.

If we are to meet contemporary challenges and prepare graduates who can provide excellent patient care wherever nursing care is needed and who can create a preferred future for the discipline, we must continue to create places for thinking together, challenging our assumptions, and envisioning and enacting pedagogies that are responsive to the contemporary contexts of care. We will not meet the many challenges we face as nurse educators by merely remembering our past or chronicling and critiquing past "movements" in nursing education. Rather, we must question the extent to which we direct our effort toward reinforcing the traditional or conventional pedagogies because we either are not familiar with other approaches or are waiting for someone else (an expert or leader in the field) to devise a solution to the challenges we face.

We hope this volume captures the spirit of the original Curriculum Revolution in nursing as much as the substance and that it inspires teachers to become leaders – to pool their intellectual prowess and long experience in nursing education to risk extending their grassroots efforts at reform and innovation into a national movement and robust science of nursing education.

References

Curriculum revolution: Mandate for change (1988). New York: National League for Nursing.

Curriculum revolution: Reconceptualizing nursing education (1989). New York: National League for Nursing.

Curriculum revolution: Redefining the student teacher relationship (1990). New York: National League for Nursing.

Curriculum revolution: Community building and activism (1991). New York: National League for Nursing Press.

Diekelmann, N. L. (2001). Narrative pedagogy: Heideggerian hermeneutical analyses of lived experiences of students, teachers, and clinicians. *Advances in Nursing Science, 23*(3), 53-71.

Falk-Rafael A. R., Chinn P. L., Anderson M. A., Laschinger, H., & Rubotzky A. M. (2004). The effectiveness of feminist pedagogy in empowering a community of learners. *Journal of Nursing Education, 43,* 107-115.

Ironside, P. M. (2004). "Covering content" and teaching thinking: Deconstructing the additive curriculum. *Journal of Nursing Education, 43,* 5-12.

Ironside, P. M. (2006). Reforming nursing education using Narrative Pedagogy: Learning and practicing interpretive thinking. *Journal of Advanced Nursing, 55,* 478-486.

Notter, L, & Robey, M. (Eds.). (1974). *Proceedings of the National League for Nursing Open Curriculum Conference I.* New York: National League for Nursing.

Notter, L., & Robey, M. (Eds.). (1975a). *Proceedings of the National League for Nursing Open Curriculum Conference II.* New York: National League for Nursing.

Notter, L., & Robey, M. (Eds.). (1975b). *Proceedings of the National League for Nursing Open Curriculum Conference III.* New York: National League for Nursing.

Notter, L., & Robey, M. (Eds.). (1976). *Proceedings of the National League for Nursing Open Curriculum Conference IV.* New York: National League for Nursing.

Notter, L., & Robey, M. (1979). *The open curriculum in nursing education: Final report of the NLN open curriculum study.* New York: National League for Nursing.

Curriculum Revolution:
A Theoretical and Philosophical Mandate for Change[1]

Nancy L. Diekelmann

A curriculum revolution is only possible if true alternatives in nursing education are explored at both the curricular and the instructional level and if the accreditation process of nursing is reexamined. The model currently used in nursing education is the one that Tyler (1950) proposed several decades ago. Two alternative models also exist: phenomenological models and critical models. In this chapter, I will discuss these models, giving particular attention to one recently developed model, Curriculum as Dialogue and Meaning (Diekelmann, 1988b), which was formulated in an attempt to meet some of the challenges that remain to be addressed in nursing education. I will also consider some of the recommendations that have been made regarding the testing and implementation of these new curricular and instructional approaches, as well as the influence of our present accreditation process on their application. Perhaps a procedure should be established that would allow schools of nursing to petition for modification of the National League for Nursing's accreditation guidelines, so that they could explore new curricular alternatives without losing their accreditation or being put on warning. In any case, whether such a procedure is created or not, it is urgent that nursing educators and administrators find ways of working together to orchestrate a curriculum revolution.

The world of curriculum and curricular models abounds in feelings of frustration and futility. Today, however, another feeling presides. It is based on the recognition that the present curricular model is but one of the many models that can be used to organize nursing education. Disillusionment with the development and administration of nursing curricula is thus gradually being supplanted by excitement and new understanding as alternatives are developed.

The educational research of the curriculum reconceptualists, such as Apple (1979, 1982, 1986), Kliebard (1977, 1987), and Pinar (1975), makes it clear that there are two fundamental questions of curriculum that must be addressed by all models, new as well as old: How should the knowledge (subject matter) that nurses need to enter nursing practice safely be selected and sequenced? What is the role of experience in nursing education? It is also clear, however, that teachers, students, clinicians, nursing knowledge, and nursing practice all constantly change. Accordingly, the new curricular models approach schooling as a process in which the essential questions are constantly being asked and no answer is considered final. From this point of view, it is impossible to say that educators have "failed" when the curriculum is changed or modified every semester or every time a course is taught. If the curriculum is developed and organized according to a process model, it is continually scrutinized and adapted to meet the ever-changing nature of nursing practice.

1. Originally published in *Curriculum revolution: Mandate for change* (1988, pp. 137-157). New York: National League for Nursing Press. Reprinted with permission.

Besides being practical, helpful, and efficient, curricular models should be flexible and allow for frequent change. The alternative models that have been proposed are less elaborate, appear to be less scientific, and require less attention to detail than the traditional model. Like creativity itself, they are not definite: they are guides rather than recipes. In what follows, I will begin with a brief discussion of the model in current use, focusing on some of its limitations, then proceed to a discussion of viable alternatives.

The Tyler Model

The Tyler model (1950), which continues to be the standard for nursing education, provides the framework for NLN accreditation criteria. It was developed by Professor Ralph Tyler as the course syllabus for Education 360, a course taught at the University of Chicago in 1949. Over time, this document has come to pervade the thoughts of teachers to such an extent that it is difficult for us even to reexamine and reevaluate some of its central features, much less change it substantially or replace it.

The Tyler framework rests on four central questions:

1. What educational purposes should the school seek to attain?

2. What educational experiences can be provided that are likely to attain these purposes?

3. How can these educational experiences be effectively organized?

4. How can we determine whether these purposes are being attained?

Most commonly, these questions are considered to make up a four-step process comprising (1) statement of objectives, (2) selection of experiences, (3) organization of experiences, and (4) evaluation. The Tyler model is a linear means-ends process whose commonsense appeal conceals the taken-for-granted assumptions of an instrumentalist view of education.

Eisner (1985) provides a good description of the scientific and technical orientation of the Tyler framework:

> The scientific and technological orientation to curriculum is one that is preoccupied with the development of means to achieve prespecified ends. Those working from this orientation tend to view schooling as a complex system that can be analyzed into its constituent components. The problem for the educator or educational technologist is to bring the system under control so that the goals it seeks to attain can be achieved. (p. 44)

The Tyler model places high value on effectiveness, efficiency, certainty, and predictability, and it emphasizes individualism and competition. It assumes that knowledge consists of facts, generalizations, principles, laws, and theories, and that things can virtually always be explained by giving causal, functional, hypothetical, or deductive reasons. It also assumes that knowledge can be directly and easily translated into specific behaviors, and it emphasizes future outcomes while deemphasizing the "here and now." Furthermore, the model does not fully explain how teachers can decide which objectives to include in the curriculum and which to leave out; instead, it appeals to consensus and proposes the "common judgment of thoughtful men and women" as its criterion.

The Tyler model has numerous good points. For one, it requires teachers to expend a great deal of time and effort on deciding what will become subject matter for the nursing curriculum. Discussion of subject matter and the role of experience in nursing education are enhanced when teachers must specify both classroom and clinical objectives in great detail. Furthermore, the technical model of nursing education has been crucial in bringing nursing curricula out of hospitals and into almost every major university in the country within the space of 25 years. That was a major accomplishment on the part of those nurse educators of the 1960s, who fought to legitimize nursing education and who were better grounded in the Tylerian model than most schools of education at the time. Some schools have developed exemplary nursing curricula based on the Tyler model and are expert at behavioral education.

Overall, the Tyler model has served us well to this point. Those schools in which this model works and is meaningful should not change simply for the sake of changing. But just as we must reconsider and revise our curricula periodically to take into account changes in students, faculty, clinical practice, and nursing knowledge, so must we also reconsider and, if necessary, revise the model on which the curricula are based. We must take advantage of the research in public education over the last 15 years and begin to consider alternative models.

The same model is used for accreditation as for instruction. It has many limitations, but here I will only mention one: the amount of time that the Tyler model forces nurse educators to spend on developing course and curriculum materials solely for the purpose of an accreditation visit. The model demands constant updating of these materials at a time when decisions about what to include and exclude from the curriculum are becoming more and more difficult to make. More than a few nurse educators are frustrated by having to prepare objectives solely because they are required, not because they are regularly used with students. For example, if at the end of the course a particular student receives a grade that seems unfair, the tool is adjusted on the basis of the objectives and the final grade reflects what the teacher thinks is fair. Some instructors spend hours using clinical tools in an effort to be fair in grading students, when this time would be better spent reading and improving their own understanding of what they are teaching. The Tyler model has encouraged educators to focus on evaluation and data gathering and to use most of their time on clinical units in evaluating students. Likewise, faculty members spend most of their energies trying to organize the curriculum. It is time to explore some alternatives.

A Quest for Alternative Orientations

The curricular literature of the 1970s reflected an interest in reconceptualizing the field of curriculum, exploring alternative paradigms or ideologies within which curriculum thought is embedded, and, most particularly, transcending behaviorism in curricular thought to embrace beingness and critical thought. Schools began to be viewed as places engaged in a search for situational meaning. During this time, the work of Eisner and Vallance (1974), Pinar and the reconceptualists (1975), Goodlad (1969), Apple (1979), and Freire (1970) manifested both a willingness to challenge the Tyler model and a desire to pursue alternative orientations. Educators must continue to explore these alternatives.

The Tyler Model as a Technical Model

The Tyler model is a technical model of education. One assumption of the technical model is that once students are given information in the classroom, they can then practice and apply it in the clinical area. Since reinforcement is important, it is considered desirable, by both students and teachers, to match a student who is studying diabetes with a diabetic patient, or a student studying problems of oxygenation with a hypoxic patient. Clinical checklists and course objectives are carefully coordinated with the aim of ensuring that students' learning is as strongly reinforced as students' clinical experience. The closer the match between theory and experience or between classroom and clinical instruction, the better and greater the learning.

A second assumption of the technical model is that all students should acquire some essential knowledge and skills. Implicit in this assumption is the notion that certain skills and knowledge should be identified by the faculty and practitioners as essential and taught to all students. Inevitably, some subject matter and skills continue to be taught even though students never encounter situations in which they can be used or practiced. There is, of course, considerable conflict among teachers regarding what knowledge and skills are essential. Sometimes this conflict raises questions of academic freedom. Schools that adhere strictly to the technical model prescribe subject matter and skills and require faculty to agree to teach the knowledge and skills identified as essential. The model assumes that faculty conflict should be resolved through compromise.

A third assumption of the technical model is that all students ought to have experience in every specialty area of nursing, or at least in as many as possible. This assumption may be operationalized as required community, operating room, or pediatric experience. Faculty, practitioners, and students alike embrace the notion that exposure to all specialty areas is essential if the student is to make appropriate employment and career choices after graduation.

Phenomenologic Models: Schools in Search of Meaning

In phenomenologic models of curriculum, the central concern is the communicative understanding of meanings given by people who live within the situation. These models (Greene, 1971; Huebner, 1975) acknowledge the possibility of multiple approaches to a phenomenon or problem. For example, it is possible to state objectives in a number of different ways, but in the final analysis it is the teacher who must interpret these printed statements and translate them into action. Instead of emphasizing the writing of objectives, phenomenologic models emphasize the processes of understanding that shape the world of the student and teacher. The written materials these models use can be identical to those used in the Tyler model; the crucial difference is that phenomenologic models of education emphasize the importance of experience and meaning.

The French existential phenomenologist Merleau-Ponty (1962) argued that a fuller understanding of any phenomenon requires a primary emphasis on how it is experienced:

> The whole universe of science is built upon the world as directly experienced, and if you want to subject science to rigorous study, we must begin by reawakening the basic experience of the world of which science is the second order experience. (p. 88)

The essence of the phenomenologic model is the attempt to come to some understanding of the world of Being, the lived world of people. The orientation is toward the here and now of the situation, and rules for the understanding of meaning are actively constructed by those who dwell within the situation.

The possibilities of the phenomenologic model for clinical education are great. In this model, clinicians develop the clinical courses in conjunction with faculty. One reason for the schism between education and practice may be that teachers feel they have to develop clinical objectives and then use them to evaluate students. Use of a phenomenologic model eliminates this emphasis on prediction and evaluation. Instead, it creates a focus on the lived experiences of clinicians and on introducing students to the clinical world. In this model, clinical nursing knowledge is an integral part of the curriculum, with practice informing the curriculum in much the same way that education has traditionally informed practice.

Teacher and student come together in the classroom, and the physical and social environment is transformed into a pedagogic situation. The essential process is not the transmission of information or the facilitation of learning, but the initiation and maintenance of dialogue. Knowing is not acquiring facts, but rather making meaning and giving meaning. To explain is to clarify common meanings and authenticate experiences. In this model, knowledge is not nomologic – that is, facts, laws, and theories – rather, it is situational meaning. This method is often used in case studies, and many teachers are at their best at those moments when they are engaging in dialogue with their students.

The phenomenologic model emphasizes the attempts of teachers-as-learners to understand the lived experiences of their students as well as their patients. To this end, expert clinicians are often brought into the classroom to lecture. Thus, teachers work with clinicians to establish exactly what the meaningful experiences – both clinical and classroom – are for students as they move from layperson to novice nurse and, for some, to graduate status. It is these life experiences within a lived situation that matter pedagogically. These experiences cannot be predicted or prescribed, but they can be demonstrated.

The role of the teacher is to seek ways of linking the contextual and conceptual worlds of students. Students need contextual rules to help them enter new situations safely. Together, teacher and student seek to link the particular with the universal; the concrete, day-to-day, personal world of action with the world of ideas, values, and symbols, or, more generally, with systems of meaning. Not only are theory and practice integrated through action and reflection, but they also constitute part of a larger interpretive endeavor directed toward the recovery of meaning and the development of understanding. Clinical courses should build on each other as students develop their expertise. The necessary link between classroom (theory) and clinical experiences is thus deconstructed.

In the phenomenologic model, the private becomes more and more public. The main goal is to understand how and in what ways one becomes a nurse. Students have considerable private knowledge about what should be validated and made visible; thus, they are considered equal participants in the development of the curriculum. As their experiences are transformed into written documents for teachers, clinicians, and other students, these experiences may trigger valuable new insights into schooling. Teaching is a way of listening and responding, of hearing and heeding what is said. Listening is by no means a merely passive state: to be a listener presupposes that one not only is in a listening situation, but also has actively taken up that situation as one's own. Teachers are the interpreters and historians who participate in a distinctive horizon of questions and experiences that throws open for students the future as possibility.

From this viewpoint, the curriculum is more than a set of objectives that serve as the parameters for the production of a nurse. Rather, it is the lived experiences of students, teachers, and clinicians as they work together in an attempt to understand how best to introduce students into the practice of nursing. The focus of the curriculum is the struggle to understand nursing knowledge and nursing practice. Caring, as an ontologic state, is fundamental to the curriculum.

Critical Models: Schools in Search of Critical Consciousness

Critical models also emphasize dialogue; where they differ from phenomenologic models is in their emphasis on a commitment to emancipation. Teachers who use these models seek to make visible to themselves and their students the power imbalances that occur in both our schools and our practice. They place high value on the critical processes of dialogue and debate, and they bring feminist and emancipatory approaches to the examination of issues confronting nursing students, both within the school and in the practice environment. Dialogue as a critical process is the foundation for this model.

Curriculum as Dialogue and Meaning

Curriculum as Dialogue and Meaning has points in common with both critical and phenomenologic models. It proposes an alternative way of conceptualizing nursing education that is based on a restructuring of the relationship between knowledge and skill acquisition. This restructuring profoundly affects how education, knowledge, experience, and expertise are defined and experienced in the nursing curriculum. In this model, the curriculum is a dialogue among teachers, practitioners, and students on what will constitute the knowledge in the nursing curriculum and what role experience will play in the curriculum. The curriculum is what it means to be a faculty-teacher researcher, a practitioner-teacher, and a student nurse. The curriculum is both constituted and constituted by these people.

In Curriculum as Dialogue and Meaning, there is no higher court for discussions than the faculty, practitioners, and students involved. Dialogue is more than conversation; it is being-in-the-world with others through language and experience. In dialogue, it is assumed that decisions are only meaningful in the context in which faculty, students, and practitioners experience them. Thus, enlightened debate in which the issues and all the complexities involved, including those of power and control, are fully discussed does not necessitate a vote or consensus to become operational. To understand a "problem" from a new perspective is to understand what the problem means. The "solution," then, is achieved contextually, since all participants – teachers, practitioners, and students – will attend in their own way to the new meanings they have experienced.

Dialogue is a joint reflection on a phenomenon; it is a deepening of experience for all participants; it is talking, generating questions, and possibly interpreting. Dialogue involves the lived experiences of everyone and seeks shared understanding. Buber (1958) describes the "between," that is, the "seeing the between" or meeting to share a viewpoint, as revealing and permitting understanding. According to Weber (1986), "it is through the seeing of that which is neither only you nor only I, but is rather our between that we learn about each other" (p. 68).

Curriculum as Dialogue and Meaning is a community of scholars, researchers, teachers, practitioners, and students who together think things through, glancing at the mirrors others hold up for them, discovering not only the other but also themselves. Dialogue is thus private and confidential, as well as social and public. It is oral discourse. Accordingly, in this model the definition of curriculum as a set of beliefs that provide a framework that guides selecting and sequencing of courses in a school is replaced by a process (dialogue) that acknowledges all as participants in the curriculum and as human beings of importance – people who understand education, research, and nursing. Dialogue is respectful, open, and responsible, and it implies a willingness to learn.

The "problems" of the curriculum are "solved" through open questioning in dialogue. Heidegger (1962) argues that "the very act of posing a question is disclosure, for to question is to sketch in advance the context of meaning in which a particular inquiry will move." The answering in turn invites more questioning, thereby also guiding the dialogue. The dialogue is thus shaped by all, becoming, for the moment, "their shared abode" (Weber, 1986, p. 68).

Sometimes dialogue permits faculty, practitioners, and students to experience the "meaningful silence" of listening and thinking, in which they may participate more through gestures than through speech. Dialogue is experiencing moments of judgment and emotional reactions. These reactions may be unspoken: one party may simply be thinking, "How interesting," or "I know how she feels, that happened to me too," or perhaps "How different from my own experience this is." Still, dialogue must always affect everyone involved, or it is not dialogue. It continues long after the participants have departed. It is often experienced in the form of recollection or reflection. "I wish I had asked. . . ," or "I'd like to know. . . ." . According to Weber (1986), "One dialogue echoes thoughts of another and through persons, ideas are exchanged, challenged, and tested" (p. 69).

Comparison of the Technical Model with the Curriculum as Dialogue and Meaning

In Curriculum as Dialogue and Meaning, knowledge is instrumental, practical, and critical. Experience is defined as the turning around of preconceived notions, or the refining and elaborating of previously held beliefs, skills, and expertise (Heidegger, 1962). Expertise is the ability to theorize using knowledge that is instrumental, practical, and critical.

As noted earlier, the technical model makes two important assumptions: that it is necessary to identify essential knowledge and skills for the curriculum, and that it is desirable to reinforce and match theory with clinical experiences. In Curriculum as Dialogue and Meaning, the curriculum is reconceptualized as containing two kinds of knowledge: one kind instrumental and theoretical and the other practical and dependent on experience – in other words, "knowing that" and "knowing how." "Knowing that" knowledge is instrumental and is that part of the curriculum taught in the classroom by teachers who are expert in theoretical knowledge. "Knowing how" knowledge is practical. It is acquired through the clinical experience of nursing and is found in the practitioners or clinical faculty. This knowledge is not, however, taught by the practitioners or the clinical faculty, because clinical knowledge cannot be taught; it can only be demonstrated. It is personal, and it can only be acquired through experience. Thus, expertise in nursing education is the use of "knowing that" knowledge to aid the development of "knowing how" knowledge in the context of nursing practice. In Curriculum as Dialogue and Meaning, the objective of clinical learning is the development of the clinical expertise of the student. This expertise is defined as the ability to make clinical decisions that take context into account. It involves clinical decision making, but in a sense that is fundamentally different from that typically captured by descriptions of the nursing process.

The objective of developing clinical expertise in students does not depend on a corresponding relationship between classroom and clinical instruction. The clinical courses can be conceptualized in relation to the development of expertise, while the classroom courses can be conceptualized in terms of the selection and sequencing of nursing knowledge. Since learning is not defined as the transfer or application of information, it is not mandatory that the student demonstrate to the teacher the transfer of a skill from one setting to another or that information in the classroom be matched with phenomena in the clinical area. For example, it is not required that students apply information in their care plans to show teachers that they can do so accurately. Thus, the elaborate coordination of classroom and clinical teaching, based on assumptions of reinforcement and a corresponding relationship between theory and practice, is not necessary.

This is not to say, however, that the selection and sequencing of subject matter for the curriculum is eliminated, for it is important that faculty, practitioners, and students spend time determining how classroom content should be presented. What is desired is a wedding of the acontextual rules of the specialty areas with the emerging clinical decision-making skills. The relationship between theory and practice, or theoretical knowledge and practical knowledge, is transactional rather than applicational. The practice area is the place where students enter into dialogue with the theories they learn in the classroom. It is through practice that theories are refined, elaborated, and challenged. Practice is theory-generating, and in this sense, as Heidegger's (1962) notions of practical knowledge preceding theoretical knowledge suggest, theoretical concerns are derivative.

Classroom and clinical learning intersect at the epistomologic level. According to the research done on clinical decision making (Benner, 1984), student nurses use rule-governed behavior to enter new nursing situations safely. The challenge for the theoretical faculty who teach in the classroom is to identify the knowledge students need for safe entry into nursing situations through the study of nursing and related fields. Today, the rules of nursing are more deeply entrenched in our textbooks and literature than ever, and the essential task for classroom teachers is to determine, through research and the generation of nursing knowledge, what rules and knowledge are actually necessary. The challenge for the clinical faculty, on the other hand, is to attempt, through research, to understand how students acquire clinical decision-making skills in nursing, as well as how they use experience to acquire nursing expertise.

The curriculum also contains what is known as critical knowledge, which is concerned with making overt and conscious the issues of power and control that affect the curriculum at all levels. This knowledge seeks to provide faculty, students, and clinicians with the greatest amount of freedom through dialogue while identifying the issues of power and control that dominate and limit such freedom within the context of the curriculum. However, the issues of power and control are never limited to the curriculum alone. Thus, the notion of "essential knowledge" is one in which all faculty, practitioners, and students have an equal interest.

Curriculum as Dialogue and Meaning contests the notion that there can be "consensual validation" of "essential knowledge." Research in education (Greene, 1971; Kliebard, 1977, 1987) showed long ago that faculty consensus on issues of subject matter tends to identify knowledge that is either obvious or trivial. For example, who would argue that nursing students do not need to know how to give an intramuscular injection safely? Consensus on this point would be easy to obtain, but it would be little more than common sense.

Dialogue raises the discussion to another level. More sophisticated questions are asked. For example, how proficient in critical care skills should baccalaureate and associate degree students be? Should they be required to develop their skill in intravenous therapy? Should mock code situations be required or optional for students? In this kind of a discussion, everyone's interest is apparent. Faculty who are generating knowledge about advanced nursing practice are concerned that students have the skills they will need to use the knowledge being generated; practitioners desire that students have the skills they need to care for the patients they are assigned; and students want the skills they need to care for patients safely both while they are in school and after they have graduated. Dialogue among faculty, practitioners, and students on what knowledge and skills are to be taught allows freer determination of classroom knowledge. Similar dialogue occurs in the identification of clinical learning experiences.

In Curriculum as Dialogue and Meaning, students need not have at least one experience in each specialty area, nor are particular specialty areas or experiences mandatory. A school may decide to impose certain requirements, after dialogue with faculty, practitioners, and students, but the rationale would not be, as it is today, that students would thereby be better prepared to select the area in which they are most skilled and would most like to practice after graduation. These choices are best left to the student's discretion.

The rationale for specifying clinical experience rests not on the job needs of the specialty but rather on the needs of the patient populations being served. Thus, it is possible to learn about caring for the chronically ill by caring for either children or adults. This is not to imply that these two groups do not have very different needs. However, if the objective of clinical instruction is to help students learn the appropriate rule-governed behavior as a part of acquiring the nursing expertise necessary to care for someone with a chronic illness, the patient population is but one variable. The provision of experiences for novice nurses that lead them from rule-governed behavior to the development of a sense of generalizable attributes and aspects is possible in any nursing specialty.

Allowing students to control the rate at which they change nursing specialty areas and nursing units is supported by research in which student nurses reported that constantly learning new units and nursing specialties interfered with their ability to enter and experience the nursing culture (Diekelmann, 1988a). The students reported understanding, and in some instances accepting, the "cold reception" they received as being legitimate, since they felt that they often did not know what they were doing and had many questions that staff nurses had to answer.

In Curriculum as Dialogue and Meaning, attention is paid to the issues of socialization as well as to the learning of the necessary clinical judgment skills. This model is based on the development of new collaborative relationships between teachers and practitioners that would allow all hospitals to be laboratories for students learning nursing, and that would allow nurses to experience as a part of schooling a caring environment in which they are valued by all nurses as a rich resource for the profession. New titles and creative use of hospital and teaching positions can make new levels of collaboration possible. For example, professor-clinicians who are doctorally prepared but hospital-based could, as part of their clinical assignment, contribute to the learning of clinical students at all levels. Placing master's students, two senior students, two junior students, and four sophomore students, all with different objectives, on a single unit could give students the opportunity to experience the nursing culture in new ways as they develop their skills and expertise in nursing. Staff nurses could be involved in clinical instruction in ways that are not dependent on classroom activities. Students could choose either to stay on a unit or in an agency for more than one semester or to specialize, which would enable them to experience the nursing culture over time.

Allowing students the option of selecting clinical experiences at the baccalaureate level is also supported by much of the research done on clinical decision making. Benner (1984) has documented that it is through developing a sense of attributes and aspects that expertise is developed in novices. To develop these aspects and attributes in a more general sense, the students must have enough similar experiences to make the appropriate judgments. For example, to learn when to make the clinical judgment of whether a particular blood pressure is meaningfully low or whether a patient is cyanotic, the student must have enough experiences in which the opportunity to make these qualitatively graded decisions are available. One way of maximizing this kind of decision-making experience is to give students the chance to [select] patient populations [during their clinical rotations].

Curriculum as Dialogue and Meaning reconceptualizes the curriculum and the assumptions regarding knowledge, experience, and expertise implicit in it. There are other important assumptions regarding temporality, being, and languages that have not been explicated but that also underlie the model.

Instructional Alternatives

Empowering

One instructional alternative worth considering is a pedagogy that is empowering. Such an approach would have as a major concern the development of students' powers of inquiry, self-knowledge, and ability to make and remake knowledge and culture. Teachers have always been attentive to the intellectual development of students, but an empowering pedagogy would place more emphasis on this process than on content (Shor, 1980). The goal would be to avoid reproducing curricula that are so full of information that there is little time to talk to students and few activities in which students think critically.

It will not be easy to find ways to have dialogue with students in today's crowded curricula; lectures do not easily lend themselves to anything besides simple transmission of information. Nevertheless, there are strategies that can be used. Language and thinking are intimately linked. The use of a variety of writing experiences across the curriculum might help students develop their critical skills. Such experiences include critiquing syllabi, not for what they include but for what they exclude. Helping students understand the critical processes clinicians and teachers bring to nursing will help them understand the nature of critical thinking in nursing practice. It is timely to explore ways of thinking about and organizing care other than in care plans, which are poor reflections of the kind of critical processes used in practice.

An increasingly important issue in nursing is the ethical quagmires that nurses are facing more and more often in practice. Dialogue with clinicians can only enhance the critical abilities of students as they enter nursing practice.

Reconciliation

A second alternative to consider is reconciliation between students and teachers to reduce hostility and to foster solidarity instead of alienation. Research based on interviews of student nurses shows that students continue to be extremely fearful (Diekelmann, 1988a). This is not a new observation; indeed, the power and control teachers wield in nursing has been a recurring theme throughout the history of nursing education. Though teachers take considerable pains to try to create supportive environments in which students can learn and grow while protecting patients and providing optimum care, novice students are still extremely fearful of teachers. Something is wrong, and teachers need to enter into dialogue with their students to find out what that might be. Talking with students about their lived experiences and their reactions to the curriculum may help create new relationships with them (Diekelmann, 1988a).

In a number of studies, students reported that they did not trust faculty. They talked about playing the game and psyching out the teacher. One student said, "What is playing the game? It's knowing what to do and what not to do, what counts and what doesn't, who to talk to and about what – that's what it is." Teachers need to explore why students are so suspicious. Certainly this will be difficult with students who have constantly been talked at and told what to do and not to do throughout their educational careers. Lack of motivation and apathy, – in Shor's (1986) phrase, performance strikes – on the part of those students should not be surprising. Nonetheless, if teachers put their energies into understanding the student experience, it may prove possible to transform their relationships with them. Teachers might then be better able to engage students in the re-creation of the nursing curriculum.

Situated Study

A third alternative is situated study, a pedagogy in which the study of one exercise merges into another. It is flexible and fluid and allows teachers to abandon the syllabus or the topic to be discussed when the students become engaged in a topic that is of interest to them.

Certainly teachers are under restrictions that may prevent them from being this flexible, but there are times when they might seek to engage students. In the Diekelmann (1988a) study, a student talks about her frustration in negotiating a paper topic. She said, "Those primary courses are really exciting to me because I didn't have any community health in my nursing program before. Like I was saying before, any new stuff is really exciting. I love it really a lot. But repetition is hard. I don't think I'm so smart that I can't learn more, but it's just that sometimes you just sit there and like you've heard it and you remember it. . . ."

This student nurse reminds me of a student on strike – a serious strike in which she is bored and unchallenged and finds the experience demeaning. Shor (1986) describes this kind of student strike well:

> Students will resist any process that disempowers them. Unequal, disabling education is symbolic violence against them, which they answer with their own skills of resistance silence, disruption, nonperformance, cheating, lateness, absence, vandalism, etc. Very familiar school routines produce this alienation: teacher talk, passive instruction in preset materials, punitive testing, . . . denial of themes and other subjects important to them, the exclusion of student coparticipation in curriculum design and governance...

The nurse quoted earlier provides a concrete example of why students strike. For example, she recalled,

> *[As students], we had to talk, give a presentation on something within the nursing field or the health medical field, and I talked about the homeless, and in my critique my teacher couldn t understand what they had to do with the health field and just went on to say that she really didn t understand what my point was of speaking on the homeless. And I had to proceed to tell her that it was an ever growing problem, especially now when people, if people don t have insurance, don t have access to the medical services, then people are sicker, people aren t seeking out the care they need. And she just, I don t know, we kind of went around and around about why I thought that was important and why I thought that had to do with something in the medical field. I don t know, I had a hard time with her. As a person, I got along with her.*

It is ironic that this student provides an example that reflects the very solution to transforming education. According to Shor (1986),

> *The vast alienation of students from school and society can drown any plan that does not empower them to transform reality, to study their culture critically and to remake it. Situated study can reverse these conditions. Any curriculum opaqueing reality instead of illuminating it, against student equality and aspirations, will sink in an ocean of rejection. (pp. 182 183)*

Many students are not used to directing their own study, so it will be difficult for them initially. Perhaps giving teachers the permission to abandon the topic to be discussed or the assignment that is required by all to engage in a meaningful topic is a good place to begin. In this way intuition, imagination, and experimentation can become valued methods of learning. Knowledge is not a fixed thing to be swallowed whole; it is invented in each class. The excitement of learning is the "making of meaning."

Teacher Work

Finally, it is necessary to take a brief look at teacher work. If teacher work is a form of intellectual labor, then how can the fundamental nature of the conditions under which we work be redefined and changed? Can we imagine a role for the teacher not as information giver or facilitator of learning but rather as learner and intellectual? Through dialogue, we could begin to do away with the widespread separation of the conceptualization of the curriculum, the planning, and the design from the nature of teacher work itself. A good first step would be to reject those conceptual frameworks that do not seem meaningful to either teachers or students.

Through dialogue, all participants in the educational process struggle to create the structural and emotional environment that is necessary for the faculty to practice, write, research, and work with each other. Faculty members are in need of empowerment as well, and the empowering stories they share with each other should speak not only of how to promote achievement or advance students along a career ladder, but also how to help students read the world of nursing critically so that they can change it through struggle and community.

Nursing Curricular and Instructional Models:
Accreditation and Innovation

Given nursing education's close historical ties to the larger world of education, it is curious that there has not been more experimentation with these alternative curricular models. A study I recently conducted with Professors Chris Tanner and David Allen (1988) revealed that the Tyler model was used to the exclusion of other models in determining accreditation criteria. Thus, to explore and implement these new models on the curricular level is to fail to meet the accreditation criteria spelled out for the curriculum. Although the criteria were not intended to make innovation and research on alternative curricular models impossible, their effect is restrictive nonetheless.

Lack of funding for educational research has also made large nursing curriculum research programs impossible. Given that declining enrollments have created a nursing shortage and students who enter nursing curricula are also consumers of educational programs, it seems obvious that research on alternatives in nursing education is urgently needed. Many innovative programs have already been initiated. In some, educators are using only a few innovative approaches; in others, they are fighting for full accreditation for their innovative curricula.

What is needed is dialogue and increased interest in exploring and researching these new approaches in nursing. Entry into practice, whether or not it will ever be formally passed, has made many nurses realize that they should consider getting baccalaureate degrees. These students are coming back to nursing schools, and curricula must be developed to meet their needs; if this is not done, they will spread the word that nothing has really changed in nursing education. All the effort that has been put into increasing the educational levels of nurses will have been wasted. Research and exploration of curricular models for RN students are desperately needed. One such alternative model is the RN-to-MS program.

It is still believed in many circles that educational research is not nursing research. Assistant professors are encouraged to develop clinical nursing research programs so that they can meet tenure criteria. Often, nurses obtain their PhD in education, but find that when they return to schools of nursing, they are forced to develop research programs [focusing on clinical issues] in nursing rather than in nursing education in order to obtain funding. The widespread view of educational research as nonscholarly and dominated by evaluation studies must be reevaluated. The Society for Research in Nursing Education needs members and support in order to raise the visibility of scholarly research in nursing education and to increase pressure to restore funding for nursing education. [The Society for Research in Nursing Education was a group supported by the NLN in 1988, when this chapter was written, is now the Nursing Education Research Advisory Council.]

It may be that teachers are discouraged because they seem to be reinventing the wheel when they try to revise curricula. They have been sold many "true alternatives" that were really nothing more than variations on the Tyler model. As a result, they have begun to ask themselves whether any real alternatives exist. Many of us remember when instructional technology was going to revolutionize education. Today, however, the era of the "talking heads" has come and gone, and educators are faced with yet another curriculum revolution. What is different about this revolution is that the questions are the same, but there is no attempt to dictate the outcome. The selection and sequencing of subject matter and the role of experience in education are basic questions; what is different now is that the curriculum is considered to be a process that often brings teachers, students, and clinicians together to talk about these questions. The curriculum should change often, because students, teachers, and clinical practices change, as does nursing knowledge itself. Thus, the struggle to develop a set of criteria that will guide the process is replaced with a series of questions that teachers will always struggle with and that will be answered differently in different contexts.

Teachers must acknowledge their lived experiences with the technical model and try to evaluate, through dialogue, just how fruitful it has been. For example, would educators labor endlessly over objectives if they were not required? Would they spend as much time discussing the framework of the curriculum in curriculum meetings if that were not a part of accreditation? Is there any evidence that well-written and tightly constructed curricula produce excellence in schools of nursing? What actually contributes to excellence in schools of nursing? Is it time for educators to enter into dialogue about the meaningful and meaningless activities they engage in as teachers? Would the one hour a day spent doing clinical evaluations be better spent talking with students? Research on the accreditation process in nursing is desperately needed. Discussion of the assets and limitations of the technical model will help teachers begin to explore other possibilities while grounding them in nursing history. Perhaps pilot projects similar to the open curriculum projects initiated during the 1970s should be started across the country to encourage exploration of alternative curricular models and alternative accreditation criteria (Notter & Robey, 1979).

Transcending Behaviorism and Instrumentalism in Curriculum Orientation

Once again, it is absolutely essential that educators have dialogue about alternatives in nursing curricula if they are to take advantage of the new possibilities that are rising in the current curriculum revolution. They must also have dialogue regarding changes in the accreditation process. Perhaps pilot schools across the country could petition for suspension of the NLN accreditation criteria and replacement of these criteria with criteria and a process that would allow the schools to experiment with new curricular models without being put on warning. Most of all, educators must continue to talk with colleagues who fought diligently to bring the technical model into nursing and into accreditation to ensure that errors are not made. These collegial voices will help others understand what it means to make fundamental changes in nursing education. Educators should learn from Professor Tyler, whose "new" model for the curriculum now enslaves us, and be wary of all new models, including such alternatives as Curriculum as Dialogue and Meaning. In conclusion, it is time for us as educators to revisit our curricular and instructional models and struggle with the fundamental question of how best to school men and women into nursing practice.

References

Apple, M. (1979). *Ideology and curriculum*. London: Routledge & Kegan Paul.

Apple, M. (Ed.). (1982). *Cultural and economic reproduction in education*. London: Routledge & Kegan Paul.

Apple, M. (1986). *Teachers and texts*. London: Routledge & Kegan Paul.

Benner, P. (1984). *From novice to expert: Excellence and power in clinical nursing practice*. Menlo Park, CA: Addison-Wesley.

Buber, M. (1958). *I and thou* (R. G. Smith, Trans.). New York: Scribner's. (Original work published 1937)

Diekelmann, N. L. (1988a). *From layperson to novice nurse: The lived experiences of nursing students*. Unpublished manuscript, School of Nursing, University of Wisconsin, Madison.

Diekelmann, N. L. (1988b). *The curriculum as dialogue and meaning*. Unpublished manuscript, School of Nursing, University of Wisconsin, Madison.

Eisner, E. (1985). *The educational imagination: On design and evaluation of school programs*. New York: Macmillan.

Eisner, E., & Vallance E. (1974). *Conflicting conceptions of curriculum*. Berkeley, CA: McCutchan.

Freire, P. (1970). *Pedagogy of the oppressed*. New York: Herder and Herder.

Goodlad, J. (1969). Curriculum: State of the field. *Review of Educational Research, 39*, 367-388.

Greene, M. (1971). Curriculum and consciousness. *Teachers College Record, 73*(2), 253-269.

Heidegger, M. (1962). *Being and time* (J. Macquarrie & E. Robinson, Trans.). New York: Harper & Row. (Original work published 1927)

Huebner, D. (1975). The tasks of the curricular theorist. In W. Pinar (Ed.), *Curriculum theorizing: The reconceptualists*. Berkeley, CA: McCutchan.

Kliebard, H. (1977). The Tyler rationale. In W. Pinar (Ed.), *Curriculum and evaluation* (pp. 56-67). Berkeley, CA: McCutchan.

Kliebard, H. (1987). *The struggle for the American curriculum, 1893 1958*. London: Routledge & Kegan Paul.

Merleau-Ponty, M. (1962). *The phenomenology of perception* (C. Smith, Trans.). Atlantic Highlands, NJ: Humanities Press. (Original work published 1945)

Notter, L., & Robey, M. (1979). *The open curriculum in nursing education: Final report of the NLN open curriculum study*. New York: National League for Nursing.

Pinar, W. (Ed.). (1975). *Curriculum theorizing: The reconceptualists*. Berkeley, CA: McCutchan.

Shor, I. (1980). *Critical teaching and everyday life*. Chicago: University of Chicago Press.

Shor, I. (1986). *Culture wars: Schools and society in the conservative restoration, 1969 1984*. London: Routledge & Kegan Paul.

Tanner, C. A., Diekelmann, N. L., & Allen, D.G. (1988). *The National League for Nursing criteria for appraisal of baccalaureate programs: A critical hermeneutical analysis*. New York: National League for Nursing.

Tyler, R. (1950). *Basic principles of curriculum and instruction*. Chicago: University of Chicago Press.

Weber, S. (1986). The nature of interviewing. *Phenomenology & Pedagogy, 4*(2), 65-70.

Recalling the Curriculum Revolution:
Innovation with Research[1]

Nancy L. Diekelmann, Pamela M. Ironside and Jennie Gunn

As *Nursing Education Perspectives* celebrates its 25th anniversary, it is important to revisit the Curriculum Revolution as a historic movement. Between 1989 and 1994, the National League for Nursing held four conferences that led to the publication of journal articles and a series of books that are thought provoking, substantive, and continue to be widely cited. This conversation, presented in part at the April 2003 NLN conference "Exploring New Pedagogies: Creating a Science for Nursing Education," involves a nursing teacher scholar, an elder scholar, and a nurse sage. Its purpose is to chronicle some of the experiences of the NLN's Curriculum Revolution and give life to a hermeneutical analysis of themes reflected in a series of manuscripts in the Curriculum Revolution series. It documents the authors' experiences and research in Narrative Pedagogy, the first nursing pedagogy from nursing research for nursing education. By revisiting the Curriculum Revolution, our past is kept before us, and the future is kept open for new possibilities.

Converging Conversations

Elder Scholar: Hello, dear Sage and Scholar! I am so happy to have the chance to talk with you both.

Scholar: It is indeed good to have this opportunity. It has been too long.

Sage: Where shall we begin?

Elder Scholar: Lately I have been pondering my experiences as a teacher in the late 1980s. I remember feeling accomplished in competency-based nursing education, using objectives to guide my teaching. But I was frustrated by what I was being told was innovative, like using auto-tutorial learning packages. All that entailed was learning a new strategy that really changed nothing, nothing substantive anyway. So the same problems continued.

Sage: Yes, my friend, I remember how you were discouraged, disappointed in the landscape of nursing education!

Elder Scholar: Very much so, and then something happened quite surprisingly. One day Frank Shaffer from the NLN called me to ask that I join in planning a conference about curriculum innovation.

Scholar: And how did you respond?

1. Originally published in *Nursing Education Perspectives* (2005, *26*, pp. 70-77) and presented in part at the National League for Nursing conference, "Exploring New Pedagogies: Creating a Science for Nursing Education," in Minneapolis, MN, April 4-5, 2003. Reprinted with permission.

Elder Scholar: I have to admit, I was so discouraged that I told him, "Nothing short of a revolution was going to get me to another conference!"

Sage: Then how did he convince you to become a major participant? What did he say?

Elder Scholar: He simply said, "That's it! Let's call it the Curriculum Revolution!"

Scholar: And was it really a revolution?

Elder Scholar: It was. We expected 200 people to attend the conference but, much to our surprise, over 400 people came. We squeezed them in everywhere! Obviously something important was happening!

Sage: Perhaps teachers are always reforming, and schools are always becoming. If that is so, your conference may have been a call to gather extant reformers.

Elder Scholar: You may be right. I wonder now, how we can create schools that gather the innovation that is always already in their midst and be open to substantive reform when it comes along?

Sage: What do you think was significant about the first conference?

Elder Scholar: Well, we critiqued behavioral objectives and the major pedagogy of the time – conventional pedagogy or competency-based education.

Sage: As I remember it, this critique supported and sustained some of the innovation that was risky at the time. Substantive critique in nursing education has never been very rampant, so this was a significant conference.

Elder Scholar: True. And since the NLN was a supporter of behavioral objectives, I respected the organization for leading this revolution and for gathering critical inquiry and scholarship.

Sage: I believe at the time, schools of nursing were accredited through standards that reflected only conventional pedagogy, and most schools were enslaved to this approach.

Elder Scholar: And we still may be, I might add, though now we have dropped the word *behavioral* from objectives and instead talk about *outcomes.*

Sage: Same suit, different shoes?

Elder Scholar: I think so. The major approach in many schools of nursing is still conventional pedagogy although we now more commonly refer to *outcomes* or *competency based education.*

Sage: Perhaps this conference was the beginning of the end of conventional pedagogies in nursing education. By end I do not mean a critique that calls for a replacement of – or for doing away with – all conventional pedagogies. Indeed, the alternative pedagogies are seen as a way to respond to the critique of the predominant pedagogy.

Elder Scholar: You mean, end as a *culmination*, a gathering of all the possibilities embedded in an approach?

Sage: Right. In this view, pedagogies that are new to nursing are not seen as being in opposition to conventional approaches. Rather, they are viewed as co-occurring and extending…

Elder Scholar: …and affirming the predominant pedagogy, all the while addressing the substantive critiques and making unique contributions.

Scholar: Were alternatives to competency-based education evident at the first conference?

Elder Scholar: Good question!

Sage: And…

Elder Scholar: And the answer is yes and no.

Sage: I take it the term pedagogy was not.

Elder Scholar: Correct. We spent a lot of time in the presentations and concurrent sessions putting our heads together to think about our persistent problems. And there were feminist and critical theory analyses of these problems as well.

Sage: The first conference did highlight problems and the need for reform.

Elder Scholar: So true. And problems like the additive curriculum held our attention.

Sage: Doesn't this sound familiar?

Elder Scholar: All too much so. There remains too much content in the nursing curriculum!

Sage: Perhaps innovation *as* overcoming problems belongs to a certain kind of thinking – analytical or metaphysical thinking.

Elder Scholar: Then every pedagogy carries with it a particular philosophy of science, or way of viewing things like knowledge, knowing, and thinking.

Sage: Excellent point! And outcomes education – conventional pedagogy – privileges analytical thinking, scientific rationality, theory, and empirical knowledge. It is particularly responsive to identifying problems that are within or created by this approach. Perhaps other pedagogies are needed now that make thinking co-equal with content presentation.

Elder Scholar: Sadly, I cannot say that alternative pedagogies – critical, feminist, phenomenological, and postmodern – were present then. They were not. In fact, I did not discover Narrative Pedagogy, our first nursing pedagogy in the United States, until 1995. This pedagogy emerged from nursing research for nursing education that was inspired by the Curriculum Revolution – it took time to develop substantive research to address these issues.

Sage: You are right. And, although the new pedagogies are more common in nursing education today, we are still deeply committed to outcomes education. Sometimes I think we are working hard to save it.

Elder Scholar: Your point is a good one. It may have reached its culmination. The problems we have now are not the kinds that are best addressed by conventional pedagogy.

Scholar: Yet we keep trying to solve our contemporary problems within the same pedagogy.

Elder Scholar: Correct. And the additive curriculum is a good example. Rather than seeking pedagogies to help us explore and address this problem, many schools continue to add more content to their curriculum to "stay current."

Sage: Then what is the solution?

Elder Scholar: Well, the solution, proposed by the American Association of Colleges of Nursing – to identify the "essentials" – has not helped the problem.

Sage: Because this solution remains within conventional pedagogy.

Elder Scholar: That's right. We need excellence in outcomes education, but we must also understand the problems this approach creates and seek out other pedagogies to address issues like the additive curriculum.

Sage: It is possible that the critiques initiated in the first conference have changed nothing, and the Curriculum Revolution has been a failure.

Elder Scholar: Certainly it encouraged teachers to talk about reform. Maybe it even legitimized the need for reform and convinced some faculty that reform was necessary. In fact, many of the presentations showed the limitations of what we now call outcomes education as well as its contributions.

Sage: But the additive curriculum?

Elder Scholar: The additive curriculum has not gone away. In fact, as we work to incorporate the explosion of biomedical knowledge into our curricula, it is worse than ever.

Was the Curriculum Revolution a Failure?

Scholar: I began my career in nursing education in the early 1990s. One of the first books I read after I accepted my first teaching job was *Curriculum Revolution: Mandate for Change.* At that time, having come to education right out of an administrative position, I had no formal preparation in teaching and no knowledge of the current educational literature.

Elder Scholar: Did you struggle to comprehend the ideas of those revolutionaries?

Scholar: Yes, but it felt right for me – it spoke to me.

Elder Scholar: And excited you?

Scholar: Exactly. It demanded my attention and convinced me that nursing education could be different from what I had experienced as a student. I know the danger in teaching as we were taught! Perhaps reading this literature "cold" was the best thing for my teaching career, because I didn't put my energies into learning the more traditional methods only to be forced to unlearn them or overcome them.

Elder Scholar: You didn't feel as if you were taking a risk?

Scholar: Absolutely! But because I was new, no matter *what* I did I was taking a risk. So I just jumped in! I tried and experimented, all the while reading everything I could get my hands on. You might say that one of the biggest contributions of the Curriculum Revolution was *to call out* a whole new generation of teachers to envision a new nursing education while also challenging current faculty. How could that be considered a failure? Haven't you witnessed a change in the new generation of teachers?

Elder Scholar: Indeed I have! But there is also a new generation of students! This fall, I was discussing with master's and doctoral students their experiences as teacher assistants in their teaching practica. One student told me about her experiences as a guest lecturer in an undergraduate course with 70 students. The course professor met with her before the class to review the objectives and the readings. She told her how she usually presents the content and even gave her a copy of her PowerPoint slides. The student, however, conducted the class differently. She asked a series of thoughtful questions, such as "What would you do if?" and she encouraged students to guess if they did not know the correct thing to do.

Scholar: So she was making the point that these students need to learn how to figure things out.

Elder Scholar: Precisely! And that meant working with each other and trying to guess when they did not know what to do. I was impressed by how easily this graduate student, who had never taught before, used several of the new pedagogies in giving her first guest lecture. I asked her about how the professor responded. She said her evaluations were excellent and the professor was amazed, saying "They got the content and *you didn't lecture a minute!*

Scholar: Did the professor ask how it was done?

Elder Scholar: Yes, and then the student realized that the professor only knew conventional pedagogies, so she told her about the exciting things you can come up with when you start thinking with the new pedagogies. She smiled as she told me, "I gave her a pile of readings and said, let's go for coffee next week and we can talk more!"

Scholar: She had enticed her professor to continue learning?

Elder Scholar: Precisely! The graduate student told us that this teacher was not current in her practice of teaching and needed to do something about it. When I asked her what this experience meant to her as a new teacher, she said, "I realize that when I think about teaching a class, I *never* think about using outcomes education unless I can't come up with any other way to teach! I realized a lot of teachers are having trouble in their classrooms, and it is not because they are not trying hard as I once believed…"

Scholar: …or are personally not good at teaching.

Elder Scholar: True. This graduate student realized the problem was that many teachers do not know better – they do not know any alternatives.

Scholar: No wonder they are having problems!

Elder Scholar: We know in nursing how important it is to keep up with the research. Yet, these alternative pedagogies in higher education have been around for over 20 years. So you are right, dear friend. At that very moment, I understood the meaning and significance of the Curriculum Revolution for today.

Scholar: So, the graduate student is at home in both outcomes education and the alternative pedagogies!

Elder Scholar: Yes, and I expect we will see amazing changes in nursing education in the next few years. In many ways the revolution has been a long one and often times invisible. But for me, this student's comments indicate that the revolution is continuing and has now entered schools of nursing with new teachers – and these teachers will join teachers like you and me to move reform forward.

Scholar: Splendid!

The Curriculum Revolution: A Grassroots Movement – One Teacher at a Time

Sage: If teaching and learning are viewed as practices that are situated in particular contexts, then they are always becoming. These practices change or do not change over time, but not changing is a kind of changing. You have described how part of reforming is being open to new ideas and new research. You have also have shown how alternative pedagogies can influence teaching practice. Are you suggesting, then, a new approach to reform?

Elder Scholar: With conventional pedagogy, reform is often from the top down; that is, curricular reform is thought to precede instructional reform. Is it reasonable to compare this new approach to reform to a grassroots revolution that takes place from the bottom up?

Scholar: Yes. And it's possible that this grassroots movement will take place one teacher at a time. When I first started teaching, I was captivated by the challenges in nursing education and by love for nursing students, so I pursued a doctorate in nursing with an emphasis in nursing education. I studied the educational literature both within and outside the discipline and became increasingly convinced that many of the alternative pedagogies held great promise for nursing education. But my first teaching position after earning my doctorate was in a small liberal arts college with a very sound nursing program – it was tried and true and graduates were doing well.

Sage: You found yourself in a fortunate position and yet…

Scholar: …yet, I had all these new pedagogies I wanted to try.

Sage: And did you?

Scholar: I did, but being new, I kept a very low profile. I didn't announce to the world how I was challenging outcomes education and trying something new. Besides, I was too busy as a new faculty member to try to convince everyone else to change.

Sage: Were the changes you have been speaking about noticeable?

Scholar: Yes and no. While I didn't talk a lot about what I was doing or try to convince my peers that this was the way we should go, the students did! They began asking all of us hard questions, and many things started changing.

Sage: Was it the type of revolution you anticipated?

Scholar: No. I anticipated it would require a total overhaul of the curriculum, the old curriculum being replaced by the new, the novel, and the unique.

Sage: But it happened one teacher at a time, correct?

Scholar: Yes, one at a time, each of us working within our own courses, our own specialties, and our own comfort zones. What I noticed in this school – and what I'm hearing from participants in my current research – is that this may be the nature of the new revolution – a revolution where everyone begins where they are, doing what they can do.

Sage: It means teachers – individually and in small groups – supporting and encouraging each other as they try something new.

Elder Scholar: Exactly! It's students showing us a better way and teaching us how to be better teachers.

Scholar: Yes – students, teachers, preceptors, researchers, and clinical instructors putting our heads together and asking, why not?

Sage: You are propelling our conversation in a very important direction. Perhaps this revolution will be about *engendering new communities* and creating *new partnerships* for reform. We could think about how to call out reform or mobilize our collective wisdom as an important area to explore together. And, of course, keeping in mind the earlier concern – how can we be sure that this grassroots reform is indeed substantive and not just a repeat of the same?

Elder Scholar: I am so glad you have called attention to the importance of asking what constitutes reform and innovation. It is important for us to meet and work on how we spend our time together as teachers.

Sage: You are saying, then, that it is important for us to put our heads together and ask some of the really difficult questions.

Elder Scholar: Yes! For instance, how do we know content is enough or too much in our courses? If reform today begins and continues with teachers taking a stand in what they do well – outcomes education – and from there making small changes, one teacher at a time, one course at a time, then the curriculum is always changing.

Sage: The issue is to determine how it is changing.

Elder Scholar: For that, we need communities in our schools where we talk more rather than less about the curriculum, teaching, and learning. Today, almost every school is involved in changing their curriculum – in fact, most of us are distressed when we even hear the words *curriculum committee* and *changing the curriculum*. My current research indicates that while we need to continue to reform our outcomes education curricula, doing the best job that we can, we also need alternatives. The revolution using the alternative pedagogies is going on now in clinical and classroom courses, with the door closed.

Scholar: …one teacher and one course at a time.

Elder Scholar: In my current multisite research, I am learning that the doors are being flung open! Perhaps that is why I am so excited about this long-awaited curriculum revolution. I also hear how often clinical faculty are leading reform. They know that outcomes education, even though it has served us well for 25 years, is no longer sufficient to prepare the *new nurse!*

Scholar: I wonder if too many teachers are teaching for a health care system that no longer exists. Perhaps clinical faculty are leading the way because they can no longer teach clinical as they were taught. The students have changed, the patients are sicker, and nurses have new roles.

Elder Scholar: It is imperative that students be good thinkers. They must be able to think on their feet and in new ways.

Scholar: Yes, and my research on reform also shows how students are bringing the innovation from one course to another. In amazing ways, they are actually asking for changes in curricula – changes that are incredible. We were wrong to assume that students are not interested in, and don't know very much about, the realities of curriculum and instruction in schools of nursing.

Elder Scholar: Perhaps what is characterizing this revolution is that *learning is at its center.*

Scholar: Yes, teachers who love learning, and are good at it, are being called back to learning more about teaching. And they are thinking about what they are learning about teaching and learning on a daily basis.

Elder Scholar: The struggle, then, is to learn how students develop meanings for their practice out of the experiences teachers provide. This problem – trying to understand how and what students are learning – will help *teachers be forever learners.*

Sage: Students and nursing knowledge will always change, and so must teachers. In this way, teachers both shape and are shaped by learning.

Elder Scholar: Learning was an early theme in this revolution. Faculty development, especially increasing pedagogical literacy, continues to be central to substantive reform.

Scholar: When teachers learn the pedagogies that are new to nursing, they not only learn the content of the new pedagogies, but – perhaps more importantly – they are called back to being learners by *putting on their thinking caps.* Many teachers have practiced in the field for years, but have never had an educational course.

Sage: They are not conversant with recent research in nursing education, or in higher education.

Elder Scholar: The NLN is currently calling for creating a science of nursing education and advocates for teachers to have a research base for their teaching practice.

Scholar: You are exactly right. We teach evidenced-based practice. Perhaps it is time for evidence-based nursing education as well. Don't you think this is how the revolution is continuing?

Sage: Without teacher reform first, there can be no substantive school reform. Remember, however, there is always danger in mandating that teachers increase their pedagogical literacy. Can you force someone to learn something when they don't want to?

Scholar: We know that it is impossible with faculty to require or force learning, though I think sometimes we forget the same is true for students.

The Curriculum Revolution: The Teacher-as-Learner and Engendering Community in Schools of Nursing

Elder Scholar: In Narrative Pedagogy, we have identified Concernful Practices of Schooling Learning Teaching (Table 1) that point to common experiences for us to ponder. One of these is *inviting* and another is *engendering community*.

Scholar: In conventional pedagogy, the role of the teacher is to facilitate learning and motivate learners.

<u>**Sage:**</u> …by inviting the students to learn.

Scholar: True. In Narrative Pedagogy, which is a phenomenological pedagogy, teaching is viewed as bringing one another to learning. With this approach, the teacher seeks to make the course compelling by inviting students to *join the teacher in learning*. The alternative pedagogies offer teachers the chance to become teachers-as-learners in increasing their pedagogical literacy.

Elder Scholar: That can be very challenging.

<u>**Sage:**</u> The alternative pedagogies all focus on the kinds of environments or learning communities that teachers and students engender and co-create.

Scholar: Again, we ponder questions such as, how do we, as faculty, spend our time together?

Elder Scholar: Faculty meetings, curriculum meetings, meetings, meetings, and more meetings.

Scholar: It strikes me that most of the time as faculty, we gather to either share information with each other or to discuss and hopefully solve problems that come up in our day-to-day teaching practice. What is noticeably absent from our gatherings are the discussions of our day-to-day teaching practice.

Elder Scholar: And it is difficult to know what innovative ideas other faculty may hold and practice because you are teaching while they are teaching.

Scholar: Exactly! Each in our own classrooms with the doors shut. *If* and *when* we discuss our practice, it is a solution-generating session – like what should we do about a student who…?

<u>**Sage:**</u> That is a curious thing, since those rare moments when we really think together about what is possible or ponder thoughts such as, "If it could be perfect," or, "What would happen if," are the most energizing and productive times we spend together.

Elder Scholar: Everyone is at their best when they spend time *thinking*...

Scholar: ...rather than focusing on solving "your teaching problem," if anyone dares to admit they have a teaching problem!

Elder Scholar: Of course, the latter approach assumes that "we" have a solution to every problem "you" face.

Sage: It is curious how often we overlook the political nature of "who" identifies problems to be solved in the first place. Are solutions proffered such that understanding is assumed? And, I would add, understanding according to whom? And whose understanding will be given priority in finding a solution?

Elder Scholar: Perhaps this is a legacy of conventional curriculum development, wherein the very nature of the curriculum outlines, in a sense, what is to be learned, when, where, and by whom, as well as what constitutes the evidence that learning has occurred.

Scholar: Perhaps, Elder, as the revolution continues, we are creating places for "intellectual legroom."

Elder Scholar: And for teachers to think about the questions before us and how we understand the nature of our practice.

Sage: Perhaps the new approaches grounded in nursing education will call us to thinking – thinking about the curriculum-as-lived.

The Curriculum Revolution AS Creating Intellectual Legroom

Elder Scholar: The example of meeting and telling (or not telling) our stories, engaging in *discussions of our day to day teaching practice*, is very illuminating and is in itself an enactment of phenomenological pedagogy.

Sage: Exactly. In Narrative Pedagogy, this would be called public storytelling.

Elder Scholar: Some schools are calling it Voices Day. New pedagogies show up in your thinking. Recall when you asked the question "Who identifies it as a problem to be solved in the first place?" That kind of thinking reflects critical pedagogy that attends to political issues of power and control in nursing education. Similarly, your comment, "I don't know what innovative ideas my colleagues may be trying because I'm teaching while they're teaching," reflects postmodern pedagogy. There, the grand narrative of "the only person who sees a teacher teach is a student" is deconstructed.

Sage: Challenging this grand narrative presents the possibility that new faculty partnerships may be needed where teachers could observe each other teaching, in situations other than team teaching or peer reviews.

Elder Scholar: Perhaps the expense and inefficiency of co-teaching – another taken-for-granted assumption or grand narrative – needs to be challenged. Everyone is at their best when they spend time *thinking* rather than on solving "your teaching problem." And heaven forbid you have to admit you have a teaching problem! When you explore the influence of the common practice of problem solving versus thinking together…

Sage: A feminist pedagogy is lingering in your comment as well.

Elder Scholar: Yes, in problem solving, the "one with the problem" that everyone else must help alleviate is commonly isolated from the group. In creating collaborative communities, the emphasis is on putting our heads together so that we can think together in ways that bring out the best in people rather than merely solving others' problems.

Sage: Labeling someone as having a "teaching problem" and the oppressive practices that accompany such labeling are central concerns of feminist pedagogy.

Elder Scholar: What excites me the most about this long revolution is how we are mobilizing our wisdom and intellectual talents.

Scholar: You are exactly right. *Substantive innovation might be in the office next door!*

Elder Scholar: Some schools of nursing are changing their curricula overnight by doing something simple.

Scholar: Can you give us an example?

Elder Scholar: I'd be delighted. At one school, every faculty meeting begins with a teacher being given 15 minutes to describe something in his or her classroom or clinical course "that works."

Scholar: Perhaps this simple activity makes visible our collective wisdom and expertise and creates a place for the scholarship of teaching.

Elder Scholar: True! And in this way schools of nursing are going about *creating intellectual legroom* for faculty and students.

Sage: Can you share another example?

Elder Scholar: Certainly. One director told of a faculty discussion regarding how to manage or survive with almost 50 extra students and no new faculty. The curriculum committee proposed a solution that was totally unacceptable.

Sage: How did the director respond?

Elder Scholar: She told the faculty, "Let's think outside the box. Stand in my shoes and imagine that your life depends on finding ways to teach all these new students *and to do it without any of the faculty dying! We must come together* and think about this!" She, of course, recalled this because faculty not only responded to this plea but…

Sage: …it was a *call or invitation to thinking.*

Elder Scholar: …and the ideas generated were so exciting. Now a major curriculum change is under way because of that meeting.

Sage: Superb! So you are suggesting then, that if you want to avoid changing your curriculum, never meet and put your heads together!

Elder Scholar: So true. Seriously, the ongoing revolution is characterized by local or *site specific reform.* If there were solutions or frameworks or strategies that we could import from the outside, we would have done so by now.

Scholar: Wait a minute! I thought you said we should learn and import the alternative pedagogies, increasing our pedagogical literacy so that we add new pedagogies to outcomes education and reform nursing education. Isn't that importing solutions and frameworks from the outside?

Elder Scholar: Your question is a good one. The alternative pedagogies are not like outcomes education. They are not frameworks or strategies that can be imported.

Sage: Are you saying, then, that the alternative pedagogies are not generalizable or transferable from one school to another?

Elder Scholar: That's right. The alternative pedagogies are *ways of thinking.* For example, in using a new pedagogy, the particular approach to thinking about the problem as it presents itself in that particular school with the particular group of faculty and students and resources is present and at-hand.

Sage: In this way, what one school "does" with a new pedagogy is not importable to another school. The approach to thinking is generalizable from school to school but the "solutions" are always site-specific.

Elder Scholar: My research is showing that current reform is not about "calling in the expert" and faculty "learning the latest," although there is always a place in conventional pedagogy for new instructional technologies.

Sage: Current reform comes from faculties gathering with students in new partnerships and using their collective wisdom to reform schools of nursing.

Elder Scholar: And so, in this way, *the new nursing education is creating in our schools places for* *intellectual legroom where intellectual, collaborative communities of learners   faculty, students, and clinical colleagues   reform nursing education by enacting alternative pedagogies.*

Leading the Curriculum Revolution: The Learner-as-Teacher

Scholar: Perhaps we can think of current reform as a call to return to thinking, learning, and innovation *with research*. As I have tried alternative pedagogies in the courses I teach, I'm often held back by my preconceptions of where my questions will lead and where I think we, as a class, should go.

Elder Scholar: You find these preconceptions to be an obstacle when you focus too much on how you will teach?

Scholar: Yes. The bigger question, the harder question, is how will I *stay forever a learner?*

Sage: That is more difficult than one would think at first glance. We are so appropriated by teacher-centered approaches to education.

Scholar: To understand how and what students are learning – to keep myself a learner – requires that I think differently about every facet of my practice. For instance, I now prepare for class by reading widely and trying to understand the nature of the issues being discussed by researchers, practitioners, students, and my peers. I make notes of the questions I may have and bring them to class. I also ask that students do the same.

Elder Scholar: And so you all share questions and think together – exploring thinking throughout the class period?

Scholar: Exactly! I ask questions such as, "How are we to think about this or that?"

Sage: There may not be an answer for this kind of question.

Scholar: Indeed – only more questioning. This transforms me from being a provider of information, or explainer of content, to being a learner. If I listen to the questions students ask and how they hear and respond to the questions of others, I am enlightened and I see the significance these issues hold for them.

Elder Scholar: Perhaps now you have come to understand both students and issues differently.

Scholar: It is so exciting when I can walk away from a class period – a class I've taught many times before – and be energized by the discussion. And then on the way home find that I am still thinking about the questions we raised. That's how I know I am a learner-as-teacher.

Elder Scholar: All of us are familiar with the concept of teacher-as-learner – teachers are always keeping current and learning new things and students are continually teaching us things we did not know. But what you are describing as a strategy, preparing to teach by thinking about questions *you* have related to the content and then bringing them to class, embraces many of the alternative pedagogies.

Sage: Yes. By not presenting content and "controlling" the class conversation, since you honestly arrive with no answers – only questions – you are using critical pedagogy to *decenter* yourself as both teacher and expert.

Scholar: And while this may seem to be a subtle difference, I have interviewed students who experience this kind of teaching as a breath of fresh air. A student told me that in two years of school, she had one teacher who never once stood up to teach. The student said, "This teacher came to class with her thoughts and ideas and her questions. It was so exciting that you wanted to do the readings so you could share your ideas!"

Sage: But you also describe an openness, using feminist pedagogies, to *listen* to students and their questions.

Elder Scholar: Yes. And in postmodern pedagogy, there is a concern for how teaching has been taken over by the grand narrative of the *teacher as information giver* and an educational system driven by outcomes. You, Scholar, have attempted to create in your classroom times where the teacher joins as a co-equal in the struggle to understand nursing practice.

Scholar: Yes, I have.

Sage: While you are doing this, you simultaneously use a phenomenological pedagogy, Narrative Pedagogy, which curiously gathers in your story all the pedagogies, for it reminds us that *learning is what teaching is all about.*

Elder Scholar: Perhaps that is what we should strive for: *creating communities of co equals students and teacher learners communities wherein learning and only learning occurs.*

Sage: But isn't there a contradiction here? You both talk about reform – one teacher at a time – yet we emphasize collaborative communities and grassroots reform.

Elder Scholar: You are wondering if there isn't danger in describing this as a grassroots revolution – one teacher at a time *and* characterized by the learner-as-teacher.

Sage: Yes. Do you consider this allowing for an individual focus at the same time?

Scholar: Good point! We failed to mention that learning is constitutively a community experience. Even when teachers are reforming their classes one at a time, they are still within learning communities and sometimes it is risky, with resistance and criticism lingering nearby.

Sage: It seems as though while the revolution continues, awareness of community life encourages excellence in schools of nursing.

Elder Scholar: It is important for each and every student and faculty member to work on getting along and co-creating a safe, fair, and respectful place for everyone.

Sage: Paying attention to the practices that improve the relationships among faculty and students is a concern of each of the alternative pedagogies.

Elder Scholar: But this again takes a conscious commitment to engendering communities. It is not easy, because if it were, we would have caring, connected communities already in our schools of nursing.

Scholar: Yes. As nurses we know how to help even the most dysfunctional families – and this is so important, because many of our schools have become toxic, and highly competitive, and isolating, and in need of our collective wisdom.

Sage: To return to your concern…

Scholar: Then thinking is both a personal and a community practice – a return to thinking and learning that resonates throughout my research on reform. Faculty – working together to improve the community life – and individual teachers bringing new questions as a new pedagogical approach in the classroom constitute multiperspectival thinking that reflects the ways of current innovation and reform. It is both personal and communal.

Elder Scholar: I see that you are proposing a revolution that begins fundamentally within and among us.

Scholar: Yes. Thinking as a personal practice and community reflective scholarship are central to the revolution and to innovation.

Recalling the Curriculum Revolution: Creating a Science of Nursing Education for Innovation with Research

Elder Scholar: Innovation is a funny thing. We talked earlier about new ways of thinking about reform and innovation.

Sage: We tend to think of innovation as something new.

Elder Scholar: Right. Innovation as something we've never heard of before – something shown or described to us by "experts."

Scholar: Something from outside – an idea we import from someone or someplace else.

Elder Scholar: We can also look at innovation by looking anew at what we are currently doing or envision that we do. It is often the case that we miss substantive change in nursing education because it's "what we've always done." We tend to assume that innovation will only occur when we reform the curriculum, when we all agree on where we should be going and how we should get there.

Sage: Perhaps in this long revolution, reforming how we *think* about innovation precedes curriculum reform.

Elder Scholar: And perhaps the revolution is at hand. It begins when we gather together to think about new possibilities for nursing education. In that way, the revolution is fundamentally within and among us. It will be sustained by persistently thinking about everything present and absent in nursing education.

Scholar: And now we have research-based pedagogies to bring into our schools and classrooms.

Elder Scholar: Not to mention nurse researchers who can bring expertise that they apply in addressing significant clinical practice challenges to explore schooling, learning, and teaching in nursing.

Sage: So true. But the major challenge remains – we need funding for research in nursing education.

Elder Scholar: We need multisite, multimethod studies that use controlled designs to examine both current practices and innovation.

Scholar: This cannot be done without significant funding – multimillion-dollar grants similar to clinical research funding. If we continue to compete for grants only outside our discipline, we must ask: will our schools continue to respond to the challenges of a new health care system and the nursing shortage?

Elder Scholar: …and to a changing student population and a shortage of nursing faculty with anecdotal knowledge or small, single-site research?

Sage: It is worrisome, isn't it?

Elder Scholar: We once mobilized support to find significant funding for nursing clinical research. We need to do it again! The NLN is leading with its call for a science for nursing education. Perhaps, most significantly, the long revolution is one of community building – creating new partnerships and finding the spaces and places to put our heads together.

Scholar: We must address research on teacher preparation in the alternative pedagogies in our graduate schools. Every doctoral student, even those who become clinical researchers, will take on roles that involve teaching. It is time to require that doctoral students have both course work and practica in nursing education!

Sage: And there should be a small cadre of doctorally prepared nurse-researchers who continue to lead innovation through research in nursing education.

Elder Scholar: But without doctoral preparation in nursing education, research and grants that support large research programs and tenure cases in major research university schools will be impossible.

Scholar: Perhaps, then, the end of education and the possibilities of the alternative pedagogies, along with the contemporary challenges for reform to prepare future nurses, will be the clarion call of the nursing community.

Elder Scholar: New partnerships for nursing education!

The Curriculum Revolution: Multiple Voices and Converging Conversations

Sage: You are right to bring us to the question of new partnerships, for partnerships are much more than personal relationships. The meaning of new partnerships includes a *gathering of many voices into converging conversations.*

Scholar: This revolution should not be one of a few voices "teaching" and "showing new possibilities" to others.

Elder Scholar: It should consist of multiple voices, coming together, examining the concerns we share in the contexts of our present teaching practices.

Scholar: This will provoke us to think further, for precisely therein lies the *pedagogical horizon* before us. If our dialogues with each other end in riddles rather than in answers, we have not been misled.

Sage: As Heidegger, a German philosopher, argued, "The task is to see the riddle."

Elder Scholar: To whom does nursing education belong? Who will lead this revolution?

Sage: Schools of nursing!

Scholar: Schools of nursing have historically been the domain of teachers.

Elder Scholar: True. Early in the Curriculum Revolution, models of education stressed teachers preplanning what was to be learned, how it was to be learned, and how students would demonstrate the extent to which they learned it.

Sage: This premise underpins conventional pedagogies.

Scholar: But how might we overcome the teacher-centeredness of nursing education and move toward new partnerships?

Sage: The alternative pedagogies draw our attention to engendering community.

Elder Scholar: But where are our communities? Whose voices will help us envision the new nursing education? How can we bring multiple voices to bear on reform in nursing education? Where are the silent voices of nursing education?

Scholar: In one of my recent classes, the students designed an interpretive study of the day-to-day experiences of chronic illness. Area citizens were invited into the classroom, but not just as participants or exemplars of chronic illness. Rather, they were involved in every step of the research process and became teachers of practical wisdom in the course.

Elder Scholar: Citizens were able to help you and the students, as well as experienced nurses studying to be educators, see new possibilities for teaching and understanding chronic illness?

Scholar: Yes. And the students and I were able to help them imagine new possibilities for living their lives with chronic illnesses. We were all learners – gathered together each week to learn more than we currently know and to follow the paths of our thinking. Thought of in that way, we became a new pedagogy.

Sage: Perhaps we don't listen enough to what our patients or clients think we should be teaching.

Scholar: Does it matter that there is a school of nursing in the neighborhood? And what of the voices of students? Where are the voices of our clinical instructors and preceptors? Does anyone hear them? Perhaps this revolution is calling us to let go of curricula qua curricula…

Sage: …giving up and letting grow.

Elder Scholar: What would our schools of nursing be like if multiple voices were brought to bear in teaching future nurses?

Scholar: Is it possible that our practice has become too complex for us to assimilate the uninitiated in a lockstep progression through a uniform series of required courses and clinical experiences?

Elder Scholar: Seemingly so.

Sage: Issues of power and control are challenged in experience, but the myths we perpetuate to ensure the predominant pedagogy continues its dominance are challenged as well by such thinking. I do not speak here of conscious, willful acts against innovation and reform, but, rather, the subtle, nuanced community practices that we reproduce, often unaware.

Elder Scholar: I see. For example, we worry that major reform is risky and may have a negative effect on NCLEX scores. Yet, where is the research that shows the major factors that influence pass rates on NCLEX? What does research indicate are the pedagogies that contribute most to excellence in schools of nursing? How do reform and innovation with the alternative pedagogies influence NCLEX pass rates?

Scholar: How can we identify and challenge the taken-for-granted assumptions of teaching and learning that stand before us and are invisible?

The Nursing Curriculum as Dialogue: Giving Up and Letting Grow

Sage: You bring us to a new path of *thinking* about our common everyday assumptions.

Elder Scholar: My research indicates that in schools of nursing, substantive reform using the new pedagogies often begins with identifying and challenging our assumptions. As teachers, we are so used to thinking about the curriculum as a framework, map, or guide that we forget to consider the implications that lockstep curricula create for both faculty and students.

Scholar: Explain please, Elder. How so?

Elder Scholar: Well, why does the beginning med/surg course precede the community-nursing course? Could the community course be the first clinical course? What evidence do we have that the time and effort we put into tightly organizing courses within the curriculum result in excellence in education? Can we begin the undergraduate curriculum with the research course and teach students how to use PDAs and develop evidence-based care plans and e-books?

Scholar: I see, and, in the same light, could the pharmacology course be replaced with courses on how to use the PDR on a PDA or the dangers and safeguards involved in accessing and using online information regarding medications?

Elder Scholar: Exactly! And throughout our conversation we have also been reminded to explore the reasons why this may not work. Too frequently, teachers who rely on their past experiences are heard to say, "We tried that once and it did not work," or they use their perspective to attempt to predict the future, saying things like, "That would create chaos and the students would not like it."

Sage: One might say that the long revolution is calling us as teacher-scholars to be more thoughtful in our dialogues.

Elder Scholar: What evidence do we have for many of our assumptions? How can we begin to test them in the name of innovation and reform? The alternative pedagogies call on us to become careful thinkers and explore our assumptions from many perspectives.

Sage: And not just dualistic thinking, like either-or, yes-no, and so forth, correct?

Scholar: Correct. But if the alternative pedagogies are calling us to practice multiperspectival thinking – that is, cycles of interpretive thinking and looking at a problem from every direction – where would we go in giving up our current view of the curriculum so that we could grow? I met an undergraduate history major recently. He told me about the degree requirements in his department – there was only an introductory course and a certain number of credit hours necessary to meet the requirements.

Elder Scholar: How would it be if students could select from all the current required courses only those that resonate for them?

Scholar: Well, I can imagine what the response from faculty would be if a prelicensure student never had to take a pediatric course! I think one of the important calls for us in this long revolution is to publicly think outside the box. In creating intellectual legroom, is it possible for teachers to think together about positions they *do not believe in* for the sake of creating *new pedagogical horizons?*

Elder Scholar: That's a compelling proposition. What is the nature of the courses that students would flock to and which ones would they *never* take?

Sage: Would teachers learn something important about the curriculum by seeing what courses interest students and when? And, taking this a step further, how might our schools of nursing be different if faculty could teach courses that interested *them?* Might we find that both teachers and students would be more engaged in such a nursing curriculum?

Scholar: I think so, and when I start to think about reform in this way, I immediately find myself thinking about all the content areas that I believe the students *need* to pass the NCLEX.

Elder Scholar: How many substantive ideas have been dismissed because of our fear of how reform will influence NCLEX?

Sage: Yet we have no evidence to suggest that the past or current board scores are what they are *because* we teach the way we do.

Scholar: In part, our worries are tightly intertwined with our commitments to conventional pedagogy wherein cognitive gain is privileged.

Elder Scholar: Do students who have been given the greatest amount of content perform better on NCLEX?

Sage: Our practical wisdom and experience tells us, certainly not.

The Curriculum Revolution: Creating New Pedagogical Horizons

Elder Scholar: Haven't we all worked with students who, while maintaining exemplary academic performance, struggled in clinical courses and vice versa?

Scholar: Perhaps the new revolution is calling us, each in our own place and within our own community, to expand our pedagogical horizons.

Sage: Is the horizon in this revolution we have been speaking about one that is already receding?

Scholar: So that even as we move toward it, it moves away?

Sage: There are always horizons, no matter how much you move toward them.

Elder Scholar: Perhaps this is the kind of horizon we need in the Curriculum Revolution – a revolution that is *never* accomplished but where we are *always on our way*.

Sage: Who can imagine calling off innovation and reform because we have achieved the perfect nursing education?

Elder Scholar: One may see failure to achieve the revolution, or arriving at the horizon, as hopeless and discouraging. This is a position that could embitter faculty.

Sage: Or, one could view the unattainability of the horizon – and the fact that there are always other horizons taking shape – as infinite possibilities. Perhaps our pedagogical horizon is not about an outcome, such as achieving the revolution and overcoming the additive curriculum, even though these are important goals we should travel toward. Rather, the Curriculum Revolution is a path – a way of living a life as a teacher.

Scholar: Creating this world for nursing scholarship assures us that we will always be open to new pedagogies as they come along. Perhaps we will always struggle with bringing in new voices and will always be learners along with our students. Then, we will always *be* becoming as we already are.

Elder Scholar: That does not mean that in undertaking the Curriculum Revolution we will not improve everything we can, including outcomes education and the additive curriculum.

Sage: Nor does it mean that in the revolution we will not make mistakes.

Elder Scholar: No doubt, we will try things that will be like taking a wood path through the woods. As you walk along together on the main path, this winding, narrow footpath calls to you, and you take a risk to go down it.

Sage: Sometimes when walking on the path you emerge ahead of those on the main journey and you have new insights and stories to tell. But other times it means stopping short when the path ends, only to join the main path again, this time behind others.

Scholar: These are crucial times for our profession, and we must be prepared to take risks for our students and our patients.

Sage: The Curriculum Revolution of the 1990s has called us together again. If we view this revolution as a pedagogical horizon, then we shift from concerns of success and accomplishments toward using this present time together to know and connect with one another in new ways through attending to our community life – the village square in our schools of nursing.

Elder Scholar: We began our conversation together with concerns about the accomplishments of the first Curriculum Revolution. We have created for ourselves a place for some intellectual legroom in which there lives the free play of ideas.

Sage: And this has led us to explore the nature of contemporary reform and the alternative pedagogies. We leave with an understanding that perhaps in this revolution, we will always and forever be – learners, clinicians, students, and teachers alike – on our way but never yet there! Long live the revolution!

Table 1. Concernful Practices of Schooling Learning Teaching
Gathering: Bringing in and Calling forth
Creating Places: Keeping Open a Future of Possibilities
Assembling: Constructing and Cultivating
Staying: Knowing and Connecting
Caring: Engendering Community
Interpreting: Unlearning and Becoming
Presencing: Attending and Being Open
Preserving Reading, Writing, Thinking, and Dialogue
Questioning: Meaning and Making Visible
Inviting: Waiting and Letting Be

Note. The Concernful Practices of Schooling Learning Teaching are from Diekelmann, N. (2001). Narrative pedagogy: Heideggerian hermeneutical analysis of lived experiences of students, teachers, and clinicians. *Advances in Nursing Science, 23*(3), 53-71.

New Directions for a New Age[1]

Em Olivia Bevis

I often cynically think that curriculum development is something one does to keep from getting bored with teaching the same way every time and something administration uses to keep the faculty busy. I feel this way because most curriculum development results in minimal changes of substance. Usually we negotiate a new philosophy or polish up an old one; we reconceptualize, theorize, and agonize some concepts and theories we want to emphasize; we integrate, irritate or deteriorate our program objectives; we switch, swap, and slide content around; we rename, malign, and design a new program of studies; we refine and realign our course outlines; and we develop evaluation tools to assess whether or not students have met the designated behaviors. Then we open the champagne and celebrate that it is over – over, that is, until a new curriculum coordinator or dean is hired and we start again. Sometimes I feel much as the great Roman philosopher/orator Seneca wrote in his *Epistles* almost 2,000 years ago: "I was shipwrecked before I got aboard."

The very repetitiveness of our curriculum development efforts should be telling us that we are not changing the substance, only the arrangement of content. In order to change the substance, to alter the type of graduate, to graduate a professional, to create a true discipline of nursing, we must have a revolution that attacks the basic tenets of nursing curriculum development; that deinstitutionalizes the Tyler curriculum model and its mandated products; that makes nursing philosophy, research, and education congruent; that distinguishes between learning that is training and learning that is education; that alters our perception of teaching and the role of the teacher; that abandons the industrial metaphor; that restructures the relative roles of classroom and clinical practice; that de-emphasizes curriculum development and concentrates on faculty development; that develops a national strategy for change; and, above all, that provides new guideposts for a new age.

I have written this paper as a manifesto in the sense defined by Webster: as a public declaration of intentions, motives or views, a public statement of policy or opinion. Its aim, while certainly difficult to realize, can be simply put: to initiate the type of curriculum revolution in nursing education described above. It will contain a brief history of curriculum development in nursing so that we gain some perspective about where we are, with a comprehensive examination of the strengths and limitations of our present curriculum development model. And, in the real sense of a manifesto, it will specify what must become our public policy in order to bring about a new age, the age of nursing as a true discipline and as a profession – policies that must be established if our revolution is to succeed.

---

1. Originally published in *Curriculum revolution: Mandate for change* (1988, pp. 27-152). New York: National League for Nursing. Reprinted with permission.

Brief History

To date, there have been four turns in nursing curriculum development and one, I believe, that must come (Figure 1). The first, which Isabel Stewart (1947) called "the first hopeful step toward reform," came in the 17th century from the French Sisters of Charity. A part of that same turn was initiated by the Deaconesses at Kaiserwerth in the 19th century.

The second turn in curriculum development occurred in 1860 and was, of course, due to the efforts of the founder of modern nursing, Florence Nightingale. Enough has been written about the school at St. Thomas that I need not belabor it here. However, I cannot resist telling you that in examining that curriculum (Nightingale, 1867) I found that, in addition to 13 mandatory areas of skill, students were required to be sober, honest, truthful, trustworthy, punctual, quiet and orderly, cleanly [sic] and neat, patient, cheerful, and kindly. (I presume at the end of this you were sainted instead of graduated.)

The third turn in curriculum came with the publication of the *Standard Curriculum for Schools of Nursing* prepared by the Education Committee of the League of Nursing Education in 1917. It was described as an "optimum" curriculum so that schools could voluntarily improve their programs.

Figure 1: Five Turns in Nursing Curriculum	
First Turn	
17th Century 19th Century	French Sisters of Charity German Deaconesses at Kaiserswerth
Second Turn	
1860	Florence Nightingale, the School at St. Thomas
Third Turn	
1917 1927 1937	The Standard Curriculum for Schools of Nursing A Curriculum for Schools of Nursing Curriculum Guide for Schools of Nursing The Education Committee of the National League of Nursing Education
Fourth Turn	
1950	Ralph Tyler: Basic Principles of Curriculum and Instruction
Fifth Turn	
1987	The Curriculum Revolution: Models Emphasizing Teaching in a Practice Discipline

It came about at a time when state requirements were minimal and not at all uniform. This book provided objectives, content, and methods for each course and listed materials, equipment, and bibliographies. It even provided a schedule for operating a school on an eight-hour plan. The objectives were not the prescriptive behavioral objectives we have grown accustomed to today, but more in the line of general and specific goals. It was revised in 1927 and again in 1937 under the title of *Curriculum Guide for Schools of Nursing.* World War II came along and so changed nursing that this book was allowed to go out of print.

It was more than a decade before another book was published that instigated the fourth turn in nursing curriculum, Ralph Tyler's course syllabus on curriculum development. However, a great deal of progress not associated with curriculum development models has been made in the time span from 1940 to the present. Not a little of this progress has been the movement of nursing education from hospital-based training programs to academic settings. As early as 1898, university courses for graduate nurses were developed at Columbia University Teachers College. Then the first real, totally collegiate school was created in 1909 when the University of Minnesota "put the whole school of nursing connected with its university hospital on a dignified standing as a professional school of the university" (Dock & Stewart, 1920). Beginning in the 1940s, literally hundreds of college and university schools of nursing opened. A second educational factor that greatly influenced nursing practice was the experiment by Mildred Montag (1951) of placing nursing curriculum in two-year colleges. In doing this, she followed the advice of several study groups (Goldmark, 1923) and nursing educational experts (Brown, 1948; Wolf, 1947). As you know, she designed a two-year course of study for "technical nurses." Based upon Montag's model, two-year colleges all over the nation developed associate of arts degree nursing programs, gradually filling the slot in the health care scene held by hospital diploma programs. One benefit of this movement was that it brought most nursing education into institutions of higher learning.

The demise of the 1937 *Curriculum Guide* left a vacuum that was filled by the 1950 publication of the Tyler curriculum development model. This, as mentioned, was the fourth and current turn in curriculum development. Essentially, this school of thought maintains that all curriculum development, regardless of the nature of the process used, must result in certain prescribed curriculum outcomes (Figure 2). These outcomes or products of curriculum development are: a philosophy; a conceptual framework (introduced as such by Taba, 1962); behaviorally defined, measurable objectives on every level (program, curriculum, course, unit or module, and learning activity); the development or selection of learning activities sorted into a program of studies; and the evaluation of learning based on the behavioral objectives.

Figure 2: Prescribed Curriculum Development Products of the Tyler-Type Models
1. A Philosophy
2. Concepts/Threads/Strands/Theoretical Constructs (conceptual framework)
3. Program objectives (behaviorally defined and measurable)
4. Level objectives (behaviorally defined and measurable)
5. Program of studies
6. Course objectives (behaviorally defined and measurable)
7. Unit or Module objectives (behaviorally defined and measurable)
8. Learning activity objectives (behaviorally defined and measurable)
9. Behaviorally defined and measurable criteria for student evaluation

The authorities may vary in their definition of curriculum, the order and sequence of the prescribed developmental steps, and the components or the content of the development steps; but they all agree on the above products.

In 1955, Ole Sand published the report of three years of action research in curriculum revision conducted at the University of Washington School of Nursing. This book substantiated the practicality of using the Tyler rationale to develop nursing curriculum. Since Ralph Tyler was consultant to the project, it is not surprising that the methodology of curriculum development used and, therefore, recommended to American nursing educators was the Tyler model. The book became a replacement for the now out-of-print *Curriculum Guide* and the Tyler rationale gradually became institutionalized by state boards of nursing and the National League for Nursing. These powerful agencies, through the use of regulations, criteria, and the way site visitors were oriented, made it mandatory to use the Tyler curriculum development products for every one of the wide variety of types of non-doctoral programs in nursing: diploma, associate of arts, baccalaureate, and master's. The obvious consequence of this forced "sameness" in curriculum development models was some degree of similarity in the graduates. It was, and remains, very difficult to differentiate among graduates of the three most popular types of programs. While I am not willing to suggest that the mandated sameness in the curriculum development model is the single cause for this (nothing is that simple), certainly the utilization of the same curriculum development model, and that one a technical or training model, is a major factor.

There were two additional forces that affirmed the Tyler-type curriculum development products as nursing curriculum dogma. The first and most obvious was my book on curriculum development, which played no small part in confirming the Tyler-type behaviorist technical model as *the* model for nursing. It served its purpose, but it is time to move forward. The second force that helped reduce a curriculum development model to nursing curriculum dogma was

Mager's (1962) book, *Preparing Instructional Objectives*. Soon after its publication, workshops were held all across the United States to insure that every nurse educator had an opportunity to attend sessions to learn to write and use "measurable, behavioral objectives" correctly. The reverence for behavioral objectives reached such a peak (and remains there) that even their development has become formula-driven and rigid.

Strengths of the Tyler Model

I cannot join the critics that would blame the Tyler rationale for all of nursing's curriculum troubles, for it has had a positive impact on the quality of nursing education. During the post-World War II period, there was a veritable explosion of health care that accompanied the general expansion of technology and education. Nursing education entered a phase of growth in both quantity and quality.

The strict insistence on measurable behavioral objectives backed by force of law, custom, and accreditation focused the training and instructional aspects of nursing in such a way as to help lift it to a highly organized, evaluation-oriented, and regulated group that provides services of reliable quality. Along with improved laws governing schools, licensure, and excellent accreditation procedures, schools of nursing have attained a quality seen in few other disciplines. They have an unusual ability to monitor and police themselves and a sense of responsibility and commitment to the public trust that is not found in any of the other like groups, medical, legal or clerical. Tyler's curriculum development products provided the tools to be used in the search for quality, and then, sadly, they became ends in themselves.

The Case for a Revolution

It is obvious to all of us here, since the title of this conference is a "Curriculum Development Revolution," that one of the problems facing us is that nursing education is currently bogging down. It is encountering increasing problems in moving nursing further along the professional continuum. The "well educated," critical-thinking nursing professional emerges infrequently from colleges and universities.

There are many reasons for this. Bloom (1987), in his recent book, *The Closing of the American Mind*, would blame it on relativism. I think it is much more than that. Some other etiologies are: the falling quality of high school graduates; the attraction of good students to other professions and occupations; the inadequate time for providing a liberal arts education simultaneously with a professional one; and the paucity of well-educated teachers. Each of these requires our attention. Some are extrinsic factors over which we have relatively little control. Most we can affect in small ways. However, the one I think most critical, and over which we do have control, is the use of the Tyler model for curriculum development. I feel compelled, therefore, to criticize that model as a basis for my proposals for change. I believe that until we do something to abolish the use of the Tyler model as the exclusively sanctioned model for curriculum development in nursing, nothing else will be successful in moving us into our new age of professionalism (Figure 3).

Figure 3: Criticism: The Case for Revolution
1. The current model is based in behaviorist learning theory and behaviorism lends itself to training, not to education.
2. Behavioral objectives are too narrow and lack the creative energy necessary to guide the awakening discovery that must mark true education.
3. Behavioral objectives, by their nature, obviate education.
4. A curriculum development model cannot be the dictator of our educational progress and our response to the societal mandate.

Criticism of the Tyler Model

My first criticism is this: the Tyler model is based in behaviorist learning theory, and behaviorism lends itself to training, not to education.

Since Tyler-type models are the only sanctioned models in nursing, they are used for all curriculum development without ascertaining whether or not other models exist that might be better for some levels of nursing education. What is helpful to some of the technical or training aspects of nursing is a liability when used for developing the professional level of curriculum. In other words, generic education, which is the initial nursing education leading to licensure, has some content that lends itself to behaviorism and, therefore, to training. However, behaviorism does not permit education. And as one moves up the educational ladder toward and through baccalaureate, master's, and doctoral education, behaviorism becomes devastatingly limiting.

Regardless of what one's philosophy and conceptual framework state about beliefs in learning and learning theory, as long as behavioral objectives are used as the sole guides for selecting and devising learning activities and as long as they are the sole source of evaluation of student learning, the *de facto* learning theory of every school is behaviorism and, therefore, the focus is on training in the technical aspects of nursing.

Behavioral objectives as the sole arbiters of learning are too narrow and lack the creative energy necessary to guide the awakening discovery that must mark true education. Behavioral objectives represent minimal achievement levels, and are effective primarily for skill training and instruction. But they are not useful for seeing patterns and finding meanings, for enculturation into the profession or for learning the creative strategies necessary to identify, classify, and solve the problems of the discipline. They stifle creativity and provide restrictive guides for evaluations. When one remembers that under the objectives model, evaluation and grading have become the power that drives teaching rather than learning (which should be the energy source), one can see how restrictive behavioral objectives are. If used exclusively – and, again, the Tyler-type technical curriculum development models currently are the only sanctioned models – they become inhibitors to achieving the very essence of professional education.

Essentially, behavioral objectives identify the concrete, measurable behaviors that the faculty perceives as important, ignoring the students' values, interests, and natural bent. Because of the nature of the legitimate objectives, teachers cannot facilitate the achievement of goals that are not empirically verifiable. Behavioral objectives are congruent with a philosophy of empiricism but out of step with humanistic-existential goals and nursing as a human science.

Behavioral objectives by their very nature negate education. Kliebard (1970) puts it very strongly:

> From a moral point of view, the emphasis on behavioral goals, despite all of the protestations to the contrary, still borders on brainwashing or at least indoctrination rather than education. We begin with some notion of how we want a person to behave and then we try to manipulate him [sic] and his environment so as to get him to behave as we want him to.

He is correct. Further, creativity, individualization, independent thinking, criticism, reflection, identifying and evaluating assumptions, inquiry into the nature of things, projecting, futuring, predicting, searching for patterns or motifs that organize the mind, viewing wholes, internalizing paradigm experiences, and finding personal meanings are not consequences of behaviorist training. Along these same lines, Watson (1979) offers the following criticism:

> Nursing is becoming established as an academic discipline that requires a liberal arts education. It is therefore incumbent on the profession and the academic community to adhere to the purpose of a university education to gain knowledge and understanding. More energy is now expended in the acquisition of scientific knowledge than of understanding. Nursing tries to understand people and how they cope with health and illness.

> [Nursing] tries to understand how health and illness and human behavior are interrelated. Nursing education rarely concentrates on that level of understanding. In some ways nursing schools are still technical, professional schools. Many teachers and schools state attempts to develop self actualization. However, they end up

hidden, primarily teaching specialized terminology, procedures,
scientific principles, the basic content of behavior, pathophysiology,
and the disease processes. (pp. 2 3)

A curriculum development model cannot be the dictator of our educational progress and the guide to our response to society's mandate. In nursing, Tyler has become less a guide for curriculum development and more a legal code. His curriculum development products have been translated into essential components. Without evidence of these there can be no approval by state boards of nursing nor accreditation by the National League for Nursing. Therefore, if a school does not follow the Tyler-type curriculum development models and cannot show the products of these models, its graduates are not allowed to take licensure examinations and its program will not be accredited. That is institutionalization at its most powerful. Our social mandate is such that it demands care that can only be given by educated professionals.

The Manifesto: Guidelines for the New Age

Based on these criticisms, it becomes apparent that we must depart from the Tyler model. We must do more than that, but we must first begin with changing the sanctity of Tyler. In order to usher in a new age for nursing, we must work together to establish a new "public policy" for nursing. The change must occur as a totality. It must be organismic. It would be an insidious sabotage of the curriculum revolution to allow even one of our pet ideas to exist unexamined and uncriticized. To that end, I offer the following suggestions. The first will come as no surprise to you considering the groundwork I have laid.

Deinstitutionalize the Tyler Curriculum Development Model

Nursing's use of the Tyler rationale for approval and accreditation was never intended by Tyler. It was designed for use as a "guide," not as a code – laws so immutable as to make the Ten Commandments easier to break without bringing down organized condemnation and punitive consequences. The Tyler-type curriculum development products have come to constitute nursing educational dogma, creating a frighteningly single-track educational prescription that ignores all aspects of education not covered by behaviors and finite, preconceived, measurable outcomes. This has, as a consequence, a curriculum as inadequate as it is limited in its conception and its implementation. It leaves as irrelevant the large mass of learned aptitudes that are not measurable. It discounts insights, analysis, and patterns. It discards any and all joy taken by the student in the private world of discovery, in the walk alone through the peaks and valleys of the student's own mind. It ignores what Watson (1985) calls "soul," a term she defines as the "spirit, inner self, or essence of the person, which is tied to a greater sense of self-awareness, a higher degree of consciousness, an inner strength and a power that can expand human capacities and allow a person to transcend his or her usual self" (p. 46). It ignores insights and learnings that incubate in the time capsule of the mind to emerge years later like the goddess of wisdom, Pallas Athene, fully armed from the brow of Zeus, to tackle some obscure enigma.

To remain with the Tyler behaviorist, technical model of curriculum development is to ignore the higher levels of thought processes that are educative and to discard or place in peril the professionalism for which all nurses strive.

Behaviorism can produce efficient nurses on a technical level; the long, successful use of behavioral objectives has proved this beyond any doubt. It can be used in professional levels of education for those aspects of nursing that are training. What it cannot do is support the changes necessary to keep pace with society's changing demands and the natural evolution of nursing into a discipline and a profession. It has not been able to do this for a long time now, and most educators know it (Figure 4).

Figure 4: The Three Types of Curriculum
1. The legitimate curriculum – training; technical
2. The illegitimate curriculum – educative; mostly syntactical
3. The hidden curriculum – socialization; mostly contextual

Therefore, every school has three curricula:

1. The legitimate curriculum: the one agreed on by the faculty in their long sessions and debates, written into plans and sanctioned by the approval and accreditation bodies.

2. The illegitimate curriculum: the one kept in the closet, that we all know is there, that we teach quite openly but cannot grade because this curriculum of insights, patterns, creativity, strategies, and understanding does not fit behavioral objectives.

3. The hidden curriculum: the one we are unaware of and which appears in the way we teach, the priorities we set, the type of methods we use, and the way we interact with students. This is the curriculum of subtle socialization, teaching initiates how to think and feel like nurses.

So we have three curricula, the legitimate, the illegitimate, and the hidden. Currently in nursing the legitimate curriculum is behaviorist. Being training-oriented and technical, it cannot support professionalism and is useful only for the technical aspects of nursing. *The professional aspects of curriculum demand that it be abandoned.* To this end, we must prevail upon the National League for Nursing and the National Council of State Boards of Nursing to support deinstitutionalization. In evaluating nursing curriculum, emphasis must not be limited to the existence of a philosophy, identified theories, behavioral objectives on every level, and behavioral objective-driven student evaluation. Instead, we must find ways to assess the merit of programs based on the two most critical curriculum factors: (1) the quality of, or the educational nature of, the learning activities and (2) the effectiveness of teacher-student interactions for fostering education.

Rather than institutionalize another model to replace the Tyler type, we must become aware of the several models now evolving. I have developed a "Professional or Educative Model." Nancy Diekelmann has developed a "Dialogue and Meaning Model." Certainly there are others I do not know about. Since we do not want to replace one dogma with another, we must allow schools to choose or develop models that satisfy their particular needs. We must not be afraid of innovation and difference. We need only fear Emerson's "hobgoblin of little minds": a foolish consistency.

Make Congruent Nursing Philosophy, Research, and Education

Already the philosophical basis of nursing is shifting. Munhall (1982), in her classic article, "Nursing Research, in Apposition or Opposition," raised questions regarding the assumptions on which nursing research was based and pointed out how nursing philosophy had evolved along a different pathway. Her identification of the assumptions underlying empiricist research methodology could well be applied to nursing curriculum. Nursing education is also in opposition to nursing's philosophical base and, like research, has continued to be driven by empiricist philosophy. I am recommending that, as in nursing research, qualitative as well as quantitative methods be used and that empiricism in the guise of behaviorism not be the only driver of nursing curriculum. Empiricist philosophy manifests itself most clearly in Thorndike's famous assertion that everything that exists, exists in some quantity and, therefore, can be measured. Under this rubric it is quite natural that learning be defined as a change in behavior and that if there is no change in behavior, learning has not occurred.

Distinguish between Learning That Is Training and Learning That Is Education

It becomes clear, then, that in our curriculum revolution the third aspect we must change is our perception of what learning is, so that training is distinguished from education in ways that give education decisive power in the curriculum.

The development of learning theory seems to have been undertaken with the assumption that a pan theory could be devised that would serve for all learning. Learning theorists advocate one theory over another, and hostilities among antagonists both amuse and bemuse those who struggle to teach. Teachers discover very quickly that all learning theories work depending upon what one is teaching.

The problem arises when teachers, in dealing with reality, find that for some learning situations and problems one theory works better than another. This suggests that there are distinct types of learning and these types are substantively different. If one took a different assumption, for instance, that there are different types of learning, it would follow that various theories of learning may be more appropriate or relevant to one type than to another. Therefore, to begin our "New Age," I have examined nursing content and used that analysis to type learning and to distinguish among those types that are training (technical) and those that are educational (professional).

The typology suggested here assumes that type of content is directly related to learning types, and that people learn different types of content differently. A student does not memorize a list of medical vocabulary and abbreviations in the same way he or she learns to innovate nursing care strategies for a patient with difficult problems. Carried to another level, it seems appropriate to define learning differently according to the various types. (Note that I am not defining learning here.) Typing learning so that training can be differentiated from education helps teachers know the kind of learning activities to develop and the kind of questions to raise with students in their interactions. Botkin, Elmandjra, and Malitza (1979), Raths (1971), Stenhouse (1980), Schwab (1979), Eisner (1982), and many others suggest that one goes about training differently from educating. It follows, therefore, that these differences can be accounted for by assuming that there are entirely different types of learning involved.

If several types of learning do exist, then these could be used, among other things, as a means of sorting content, of differentiating between technical and professional education, and of differentiating among levels of professional education.

Since distinctions between training and education are necessary to all "New Age" curriculum models, brief descriptions of each of the six types of learning and their uses follow** (Figure 5).

> *I. Item learning* deals with learning separate pieces of information, individual factors, and simple relationships (e.g., lists and procedures), and the use of tools and equipment (e.g., catheters and monitors). It deals with acquiring the ability to complete a task mechanically and ritualistically; for example, how to take a temperature and appropriate sites for taking it.
>
> *II. Directive learning* is specifically concerned with rules, injunctions, and exceptions to rules. It deals with the "do's" and "don'ts" regarding tasks. This type of learning includes the assembling of items into a safe system of directions. By necessity, directive learning follows item learning or can be learned concurrently; for example, when and when not to take an oral temperature.

**This material was developed in collaboration with Tamar Bermann,
Chief Researcher, Work Research Institutes, Oslo, Norway.

Figure 5: Types of Learning
1. **ITEM LEARNING**: separate pieces of information, individual factors, and simple relationships such as lists, procedures, using tools and equipment. It is mechanical and ritualistic.
2. **DIRECTIVE LEARNING**: rules, injunctions, and exceptions; the "do's" and "don'ts" regarding tasks. It is assembling items into a safe system of directions.
3. **RATIONAL LEARNING**: uses theory to buttress or inform practice. Addresses why one nursing intervention is better than another. It is characterized by logical arrangements of the items and directions, addresses the logical use of formal properties and theories, and enables learners to relate information, feelings, ideas, and plans to skills. It exerts influence on judgment and decision making, and enables the learner to apply research to practice.
4. **SYNTACTICAL LEARNING**: seeing meaningful wholes, relationships, and patterns; departure from rule-driven care; providing individualized, unique client care with care models that are grounded in practice-supporting personal guides and paradigms; addresses the lived moment and the relationships that ideas, concepts, and theories have with each other; consequential reasoning and substantive views of relationships; having insights and finding meanings. This type enables people to make intuitive leaps and to trust them, and helps weld together theory and practice to support praxis.
5. **CONTEXTUAL LEARNING**: culturality; the mores, folkways, rites, rituals, and accepted ways of being a nurse; the language and other symbols of nursing; political expertise in the profession and its use; power and its use; work role relationships; values, esthetics, ethics, and philosophy. This type influences nurses' transactions with clients and with colleagues so that these transactions are caring, compassionate, and positive.
6. **INQUIRY LEARNING**: creativity; investigation, theorizing, strategizing, identifying, clarifying, and categorizing problems and approaches to solving them. It is idea generating: leaping into new dimensions; posing questions, formulating positions, fantasizing new ways, alterations that improve things and systems; projecting, futuring, predicting from knowns to unknowns using both data and intuition; visualizing possibilities, dreaming dreams, having visions, and devising ways to make real these possible realities. It is seeing assumptions that are behind positions and questioning their validity; seeing beyond words to their implications and applications and enjoying the quest as much as the success.

III. *Rational learning* uses theory to buttress practice. It provides the rationale for why one nursing intervention is better than another. It enables the learner to study rationales and the use of theories in practice. It is characterized by arranging items and directions in some logical order, and finding theories to inform practice (or, if you prefer, on which to base practice). It addresses the logical use of formal properties of activities and theories, and enables the learner to relate information, feelings, ideas, and plans to skills. It exerts influence on judgment and decision making, and enables the learner to apply research to practice; for example, focus would be directed to the physiological rationale of why a nurse would not take an oral temperature soon after the client has had a drink of cold water.

These first three types of learning strategies aid in the training of nurses and are the focus of technical nursing programs only.

> *IV. Syntactical learning* is characterized by the logical structure or arrangement of data into meaningful wholes, and will influence how a nurse uses all other types of learning. The qualities of circumstances are used in ways that enable departure from rule-driven interventions or responses and to a provision of care that is individualized to unique client situations. The use of formal and informal properties and the ability to relate experiences to care are of concern here.

Syntactical learning is finding patterns, examples, and models that are grounded in practice and that support formation of personal general guides and paradigms. It also provides the nurse with an understanding of when and under what circumstances to depart from these guides and paradigms. It addresses the lived moment; the relationships that ideas, concepts, and theories have with each other in practical usage. Such consequential reasoning and substantive views of relationships are characterized by viewing wholes, having insights, and finding meanings. It provides the reality and structure for evaluation. Syntactical learning enables nurses to make intuitive leaps and to trust them. It helps weld together theory and practice in such a way that actual praxis exists. High levels of learning in this category make the experts described by Benner (1984).

The foundations of syntactical learning are laid in generic baccalaureate programs, but real syntactical learning is seldom attained without experience or a master's clinical specialization. An example of syntactical learning would be the quick clinical insight necessary to know not to waste three to five minutes taking a temperature on a child but to move quickly to head off a convulsion that will be the inevitable consequence of a child's high fever.

> *V. Contextual learning* is the interrelated conditions in which the discipline and its practice exist or occur. It is the essence of nursing. It is learning the things that characterize nursing and make it unique. Contextual learning focuses on the sociocultural context of the discipline: the mores, folkways, rites, rituals, and accepted ways of being a nurse. It helps the learner think and feel like a nurse. It encompasses the language and other symbols of nursing. It is the development of political expertise in the profession and it is used in health agencies, in government, and in education to shape policy and legislation. It is, in other words, the acquisition of power and its use. Contextual learning deals with the relationships in the work roles of coordination, collaboration, colleagueship. It is learning the values, esthetics, ethics, and general philosophy of nursing. It is learning to perceive nursing as a human science in ways that influence nurses'

transactions with clients and with colleagues so that these transactions are caring, compassionate, and positive.

VI. Inquiry learning is the creative aspect of nursing. It is the art of investigation, the search for truth, the generation of theory. Strategizing is the main theme in this category. It contains materials that help nurses learn how to identify, clarify, and categorize problems and ways or approaches to solving the problems of nursing as it attempts to be responsive to the society it serves. Further, it is idea generating: leaping creatively into new dimensions, posing questions, formulating positions, fantasizing new ways to improve things and systems; projecting, futuring, predicting from knowns to unknowns using both data and intuition; visualizing possibilities, dreaming dreams, having visions, and devising ways to make real these possible realities. In this category the nurse learns to see assumptions that are behind positions and to question their validity, to see beyond words to their implications and applications, and to enjoy the quest as much as the success.

What becomes clear in all of this is that in order to achieve what Botkin, Elmandjra, and Malitza (1979) refer to as "innovative" learning and what the AACN refers to as "professional nursing," one must alter the curriculum in ways to promote teaching that educates rather than trains. Adding college courses and stressing rationale is insufficient. Socialization through the "hidden curriculum" is insufficient. Syntactical, contextual, and inquiry learning must become legitimate throughout the curriculum.

Alter Our Perception of Teaching and the Role of the Teacher

Sakalys and Watson (1985) reviewed seven studies done in the 1980s: the *Paidaia Proposal* (1982), *Physicians for the 21st Century* (1984), *President Bok s Report to the Harvard Board of Overseers* (1984), *The National Institute of Education Report* (1984), *the National Endowment for Humanities Report* (1984), the *Institute of Medicine Report* (1983), and the *National Commission on Nursing Study* (1983). From these and the document of the AACN (1986), Sykalys and Watson derived six curricular recommendations and five instructional recommendations. Those germane to my manifesto are curricular recommendations 2 and 4, which read, respectively: "increased emphasis on intellectual skills such as analytic, problem-solving and critical thinking skills" and "increased emphasis on fundamental and essential attitudes and values." These fall into learning types: 4 syntactical, 5 contextual, and 6 inquiry. For instructional recommendations, all four recommendations speak to the alteration of our perceptions of teaching and teaching roles. They call for: 1) increased emphasis on "good teaching"; 2) increased emphasis on promoting active modes of learning; 3) increased utilization of Socratic teaching strategies; and 4) increased student-faculty interaction in the learning environment (see Figure 6).

Figure 6: The Teacher's Roles
Purposes:
1. Insure safety.
2. Provide the climate, the structure, and the dialogue that promotes praxis.
Roles:
1. Design ways to engage the student in mental processes of analysis of cues until patterns are seen that provide paradigms for practice.
2. Raise questions that require reading, observation, analysis, and reflection upon patient care.
3. Nurture the learner.
4. Nurture the ethical ideal.
5. Nurture the caring role.
6. Nurture the creative drive.
7. Nurture curiosity and the search for satisfying ideas.
8. Nurture assertiveness.
9. Support the spirit of inquiry.
10. Nurture the desire to seek dialogue about care and be available for that dialogue.
11. Interact with students as persons of worth, dignity, intelligence, and high scholarly standards

The message is clear: To mount our revolution we must dispense with the view of the teacher as an information-giver either in the classroom or in the practicum. The teacher's main purpose, beyond the minimal activity of insuring safety, is to provide the climate, the structure, and the dialogue that promotes praxis. The teacher's role is to design ways to engage the student in the mental processes of analysis of cues until patterns are seen that provide paradigms for practice. Further, the teacher's role is to raise questions that require reading, observation, analysis, and reflection upon patient care. The teacher's role is to nurture the learner: to nurture the ethical ideal, to nurture the caring role, to nurture the creative drive, to nurture curiosity and the search for satisfying ideas, to nurture assertiveness and the spirit of inquiry together with the desire to seek dialogue about care, and to be available for that dialogue. The teacher's role is to interact with students as persons of worth, dignity, intelligence, and high scholarly standards.

In the classroom and in practicums, teachers must begin to see themselves as what Stenhouse (1980) calls "expert learners." As expert learners, their primary role revolves around helping students, as novice learners, learn how to learn: how to be scholars, how to think critically, how to gain insights and find meanings, how to see patterns, and how to capitalize on their paradigm experiences. Teachers must see their role as structuring learning activities to help achieve these ends.

Essentially, the teacher's main problem is not what to lecture on, nor how to organize that lecture. The teacher's main problems are two: what learning activities to select or design that will promote the type of learning desired, and what kinds of teacher-student transactions will best promote educative learning. Solving these two problems must become the central issues in any professional curriculum development paradigm.

To promote educative learning, teachers need a clearer idea of the ways to facilitate syntactical, contextual, and inquiry learning. Some clues can be found in examining learning modalities and heuristics of scholarship. Intellectual modes enable the learner to cope with syntax and inquiry and enable all the other types to make sense to the learner. If teachers recognize the value of these modes, they can raise issues and questions that provide the subject matter for teacher-student interactions. Such interactions would require the student to use these modes in the learning process. In the end, it is how well and appropriately the intellectual modes are used that characterizes an expert learner (Figure 7).

Figure 7: Intellectual Modes That Characterize the Expert Learner
1. Analyzing.
2. Critiquing.
3. Recognizing insights.
4. Identifying and evaluating assumptions.
5. Inquiring into the nature of things using all available methods.
6. Projecting, futuring, anticipating, predicting or hypothesizing from knowns to unknowns.
7. Searching for structural or organizational motifs or building them.
8. Engaging in praxis: enabling theory and practice each to inform and shape the other.
9. Evaluating: assessing merit using criteria and expert judgment.
10. Viewing wholes, not just parts in relation to each other.
11. Acknowledging paradigm experiences and cases in ways that enable them to be useful in practice and theorizing.
12. Finding meanings in ideas and experiences.
13. Strategizing.

Some learners will use these modes in training, but they use them minimally. However, it hardly bears remarking that all learners have insights, find meanings, anticipate, project, and structure. It is the frequency, the habitual approach, the valuing of these intellectual modes, and the expertise of their use that mark educative learning. Further, it is the types of conclusions, ideas, and insights that are derived from these modes that distinguish the educated mind and the quality of abstractions that can be elicited from them by the student.

Change Our Metaphor

The metaphor in nursing education has long been an industrial one, wherein schools are seen as some kind of factory and students are referred to as "products." Yet nursing schools are not manufacturers of nurses and graduates are not products. Products are objects, but students, like graduates, are subjects.

Words are powerful things. Speaking of people as products leads to thinking of them as products; thinking of students as products leads to treating them as objects. The behaviorist models of curriculum development are more compatible with the industrial metaphor than is a professional model. For the professional model, I suggest we do not need a metaphor. It is sufficient that we are educators; education has a language, a language of human beings, wherein people who are enrolled are called students and those who fulfill the requirements are called graduates.

Restructure the Relative Roles of the Classroom and the Clinical Practice Area

In practice disciplines, such as nursing, the curriculum plan becomes a lived curriculum within the classroom and clinical practicum. Classroom teaching is often referred to as "theory," but this is a misleading title, in that "theory" is encountered in educative teaching regardless of the setting. In professional nursing education, only theory that has an intimate relationship with practice has relevance. Theory that either originates in practice or is tried out (tested) with real people and discussed among nurses and other colleagues can grow, change, develop or become verified . . . in other words, become "living theory." Living theory does not arise in the classroom and then is "tried out" in the practicum. Nor is it the reverse, in which it arises in the practicum and is then discussed to reveal meanings in the classroom. Living theory is encountered in praxis, a dance wherein ideas, concepts, and theories may rise in the intellect from reading, discussions, lectures, classroom learning activities or in practice. Practice both tests and enhances theory, and theory both tests and enhances practice. Each enlightens the other, provoking insights, altering and changing the form, shape, and meanings of each. As the theory evolves, so the practice evolves. In this way, in the truly professional curriculum, each informs the other in the magical whole of praxis.

De-Emphasize Curriculum Development and Concentrate on Faculty Development

If faculty have any courses in nursing education at all, they come to us from the Tyler/Bevis legacy. What they know is training, not education. Curriculum development, then, as I said in my introductory remarks, just rearranges things and, if we are lucky, improves on training. In our revolution, all curriculum development starts with faculty development, wherein faculty are helped to make the transition to educational practices, to the art of raising questions that provoke dialogue and facilitate insight, patterns, meanings, and the other characteristics of education discussed earlier. Faculty development must concentrate on helping faculty alter their perception of their role.

If faculty development is successful, the curriculum will change as a natural consequence of faculty dialogue. I will not go into that here, but Joseph Schwab (1979) offers several excellent suggestions about how that process occurs. We must not equate content selection with curriculum development. Content selection is a very small part of the process. Faculty development is the key.

Develop a National Strategy for the Revolution

Without a national strategy, without leadership, there will be lots of talk and little change. Perhaps an evolution that gradually loosens the bondage of institutionalized sanctions supporting the Tyler models may occur, but there will be no great change. We must have a group of leaders to map our strategy, leaders who will give their energy, time, and scholarship to making the revolution a reality. Dreams do come true and we can fly over the rainbow, not from wishing it so, but by making it so with commitment and hard work.

Conclusion

In conclusion, (Figure 8), what is sought for nursing education is a legitimization of the educational and professional elements of curriculum; an endorsement of the dynamic, creative whole of education; a legitimization of the teaching of inquiry, reflection, criticism, independence, creativity, and caring. It must include all aspects of nursing education, the legitimate, illegitimate, and hidden curricula. A methodology for curriculum development is needed that will provide a new type of graduate, a substantively different graduate, because the planning process emphasizes the selection of experiences and the character and quality of teacher-student interactions instead of closely held, highly structured, prescribed outcomes. The graduate must be different because the values are different, the emphasis placed is different, the roles of teachers and students are different, the types of learning activities are different. In other words, the content may remain similar but the approach to the content is so altered that the curriculum itself is different and consequently the graduates are professionals.

Figure 8: Manifesto for a Curriculum Revolution
Purposes:
1. Substantively change the nature of the graduate of professional schools.
2. Create a true discipline of nursing.
Recommendations:
1. Deinstitutionalize the Tyler curriculum development model and its mandated products.
2. Make nursing philosophy, research, and education congruent.
3. Distinguish between learning that is training and learning that is educational.
4. Alter perceptions of teaching and the role of the teacher.
5. Abandon the industrial metaphor.
6. Restructure the relative roles of classroom and clinical practice.
7. De-emphasize curriculum development and concentrate on faculty development.
8. Develop a national strategy for curriculum change.

Therefore, it is essential that nursing educators and curriculum experts seek new models for curriculum development that offer a means for developing curriculum that will facilitate students in developing creative, dynamic modes of approaching nursing care. These models must emphasize the selection or creation of learning activities that promote educative learning and teacher-student interactions that help students learn syntax, context, and inquiry.

This can be done only with a different kind of curriculum development: one that provides a wider range of options, a greater scope of ideas, a valuing of active teaching strategies; one that views teacher development as the primary goal and curriculum development as a by-product; one that redefines learning, supports student creative thought as the essence of education, and has an underlying assumption that nursing is a human science.

Eleanor Roosevelt said, "We face the future fortified only with the lessons we have learned from the past. It is today that we must create the world of the future. . . . In a very real sense, tomorrow is now." For nursing education, tomorrow has come.

References

Benner, P. (1984). *From novice to expert: Excellence and power in clinical nursing practice.* Menlo Park, CA: Addison-Wesley.

Bloom, A. (1987). *The closing of the American mind.* New York: Simon and Schuster.

Botkin, J. W., Elmandjra, M., & Malitza, M. (1979). *No limits to learning: Bridging the human gap.* New York: Pergamon Press.

Brown, E. L .(1948). *Nursing for the future.* New York: Russell Sage Foundation.

Chayer, M. (1947). *Nursing in modern society.* New York: G. P. Putnam's Sons.

Dock, L., & Stewart, I. (1920). *A short history of nursing.* New York: G. P. Putnam's Sons.

Eisner, E. (1982). *Cognition and curriculum: A basis for deciding what to teach.* New York: Longman, John Dewey Lecture Series, No. 18.

Eisner, E. (Ed.). (1985). *Learning and teaching the way of knowing, Eighty fourth yearbook of the National Society for the Study of Education, Part II.* Chicago: University of Chicago Press.

Goldmark, J. (Ed.). (1923). *Study on nursing and nursing education in the United States.* New York: Rockefeller Foundation.

Kliebard, H. M. (1970). The Tyler rationale. *School Review, 78,* 259-272.

Mager, R. (1962). *Preparing instructional objectives* (2nd ed.). Belmont, CA: Feron.

Montag, M. (1951). *The education of nursing technicians.* New York: Putnam.

Munhall, P. L. (1982). Nursing philosophy and nursing research: In apposition or opposition? *Nursing Research, 31,* 176-181.

National League of Nursing Education, Committee on Curriculum. (1917, 1927, 1937). *Curriculum guide for schools of nursing.* New York: National League of Nursing Education.

Nightingale, F. (1867). Suggestions on the subject of providing, training, and organizing nurses for the sick poor in workhouse infirmaries (Appendix No. 3). In L. Seymer (Ed.). (1954). *Selected writings of Florence Nightingale.* New York: Macmillan.

Raths, J. D. (1971). Teaching without specific objectives. *Educational Leadership, 28,* 714-720.

Sakalys, J., & Watson, J. (1985). New directions in higher education: A review of trends. *Journal of Professional Nursing, 1*(5), 293-299.

Sand, O. (1955). *Curriculum study in basic nursing education.* New York: G. P. Putnam's Sons.

Schwab J. (1979). *Science, curriculum and liberal education: Selected essays*. Chicago: University of Chicago Press.

Stewart, I. (1947). *The education of nurses, historical foundations and modern trends*. New York: Macmillan.

Stenhouse, L. (Ed.). (1980). *Curriculum research and development in action*. London: Heinemann Educational Books.

Taba, H. (1962). *Curriculum development, theory and practice*. New York: Harcourt, Brace and World.

Tyler, R. W. (1950). *Basic principles of curriculum and instruction*. Chicago: University of Chicago Press.

Watson, J. (1979). *Nursing: The philosophy and science of caring*. Boulder, CO: Colorado Associated University Press.

Watson, J. (1985). *Nursing: Human science and human care: A theory of nursing*. Norwalk, CT: Appleton-Century-Crofts.

Wolf, L. (1947) *Nursing*. New York: Appleton-Century.

The Curriculum Consequences: Aftermath of Revolution[1]

Em Olivia Bevis

Revolutions Are Fearsome Beasts

Revolutions scare me. They are often bloody and destructive, accompanied by the sound of bombs and followed by the hush of silence after destruction. They are a time of noise, waste, and devastation . . . a time when passion rules and reason abdicates. They are fearsome beasts resembling the flesh-eating Tasmanian devils. All too often, the world is not a better place when the revolution is over; tyranny simply exists under another name. Consider world history and let the French la Guillotine, Oliver Cromwell, Lenin, Stalin, Mao, Franco, and Castro be witness for my claims.

Most revolutions have a few proletarian intellectuals who think they can control things. But revolutions are war, and in war only Ares and Eris, the gods of war and discord, rule. As a part of revolution, people of reason and wisdom are often martyred. After revolution there are periods of rigidly prescribed behaviors, and those who do not conform are discounted – and too often discontinued.

Given the social psychology of revolution, I prefer a longer period of planned change – not evolution, for that takes too long – but planned change. In this, we would set up tasks to be accomplished and establish task forces to work on them. Perhaps as we move toward new paradigms for curriculum development we will see an alteration in climate that will permit planned change rather than the chaos of revolution. However, for the purposes of this chapter, I must assume that we are dealing with a revolution, and I will attempt to help structure it to have as many of the positive and as few of the negative potential consequences of revolution as possible.

Construction: The Sublime Mission of Revolution

Divisiveness or Unity

As in any revolution, the revolt is not enough; the sublime mission is to construct. In order that it not be a null revolution, we must be very clear about how we know when the revolution is succeeding. Can revolutionaries disagree on the aftermath and still be successful? Or must all revolutions result in power struggles? Nursing's history is rife with class conflict. As an oppressed group with all the problems of oppression, we are always more ready to fight each other than to unite against a common threat.

We must break the barriers of social class stratification that divide us. The social status prejudices that exist among teachers of nursing spring from the same kind of ignorance and bigotry that support sexism, racism, and anti-Semitism. It is immoral and antithetical to our

---

1. Originally published in *Curriculum revolution: Reconceptualizing nursing education* (1989, pp. 115-134). New York: National League for Nursing. Reprinted with permission.

goals and we must not allow it to continue to flourish in our new world. We must value the strengths and contributions of each program so that all faculties – associate degree, diploma, baccalaureate, master's, and doctorate – participate together in shaping the revolution. Only in this way can we prevent the oppression inherent in class status from casting its dark shadow over the future. This evil carries in it the seeds of failure.

I am hopeful that developmentally we are outgrowing the factionalism that has plagued us and we can work together to plan an acceptable future. To do this we need some general agreement regarding what points of reference we can trust to tell us that we have not traded one tyranny for another but have actually succeeded in changing nursing education in ways that make us more able to meet the nursing needs of society in the 21st century. Notice that I said some general agreements. We do not want, nor do we need, rigid parameters that dictate content or process or prescribe curriculum elements.

Indicators of Success

What are we moving toward? What are we constructing? What characteristics will distinguish the new from the old? These are questions that must be answered now, not at the end, for these answers become both the goals of the revolution and the criteria of success.

Assumptions About the Future

Before launching my projections about the new world of nursing education, it is necessary to comment about some of the assumptions regarding the future world in which nursing will exist:

1. The three major sources of health problems of the next 30 years are likely to be the great increases in the population of the eldest elderly, prolonged survival of more health-threatened people that will radically increase the numbers of the chronically ill, and the growing number of people with AIDS. All three of these are problems for which nursing care is the major health industry provider. Therefore, it can be assumed that the need for nursing care will rise logarithmically, and nursing personnel shortages will continue to be an industry problem.

2. Medical science has brought us to impossible choices that disturb our deepest sense of ethics and our moral commitments as nurses. Our ability to enable more people to live out the full extent of human life expectancy has had a major effect on the strains now placed upon society's and nursing's ability to cope with the numbers of persons needing health and nursing care. As a result we can make the following assumptions:

> a. Practicing nurses must be ethically grounded and be perspicacious, wise, and compassionate in order to shoulder their share of responsibility for the morality of health care.

b. Medical science will continue to place emphasis upon high levels of technology. Nurses must not only be able to work effectively in these technically complex environments, but be able to humanize these environments with caring and concern so that clients are persons, not objects of health care.

c. The strains of aging, chronicity, and AIDS will so stress the health care system and the country's precarious fiscal balance that survival of capitalistic democracy will require a total shift in the health care paradigm. Nursing will need to assume a major role in the restructuring process, both in policy setting and in care delivery.

Implications of Assumptions

As a consequence of these factors, nursing education is required to provide society with nurses who are highly educated, highly skilled scholar-clinicians in sufficient numbers to rise to the task of fulfilling the roles ascribed by the social mandate. Any revolution that fails to be attentive to these needs will render nursing impotent to deal with the needs of society and individuals, and nurses will be a footnote to history rather than one of the main players. Therefore, the revolution must result in substantive changes – changes that alter the nature of the graduate and provide the graduate with the skills, tools, and creative thinking necessary to be autonomous, imaginative, inventive, flexible, caring, ethical professionals committed to the whole range of possibilities from national policy setting to patient care.

Graduate characteristics are a result of two things: the type of student that is recruited and the curriculum of the student's education. I shall address curriculum first because studies show that students change as a result of schooling. Note the work done on the influence of formal higher education on moral reasoning. Felton and Parsons (1984) found that education had a significant impact on overall ethical/moral reasoning levels. This supported previous research findings reported by Rest (1979) that education is a significant variable in the development of ethical/moral reasoning. In addition, the research revealed that neither socioeconomic level nor years of work experience were significantly related to ethical and moral reasoning. Furthermore, the findings indicated that stabilization of ethical/moral development occurs at the point one leaves formal education and that the educational experience may counteract moral and ethical reasoning that is influenced by work experience. One might surmise that ethical and moral reasoning would be the most difficult aspect of adults to alter, but these two studies indicate that this is not true and that education has a significant impact.

If it is true of ethical and moral reasoning, it follows that it is probably true of other important characteristics. Certainly the Edwards Personal Preference Inventory I used in two very different baccalaureate programs to determine changes in student characteristics during their nursing education showed definitive shifts in several areas.

Therefore, I shall first take as indicators of success, curriculum factors that find some agreement among those of my colleagues who are outspoken in their support of the curriculum revolution. Then I will look to other areas.

Criteria Based on Apparent Agreement

I think it important to note here that educators working on new paradigms for curriculum development in nursing are in agreement about some general directions. Some of these may be the material from which indicators of success are drawn.

One of these common agreements is basic to the whole paradigm shift that this revolution is about. It is something I hold as first principle (not as criteria): that any and all changes in the paradigm must in some way affect the liberation and empowerment of people – both students and teachers. It is an indisputable theme in our revolution literature, in our discussion groups, and in our examples.

I raise the question: Is power of limited quantity so that when I empower others (students), I disempower myself? Or is power, like love, of unlimited quantity, so that the more I share, the more I have. And through empowering others, I also empower myself. I am attempting to think, not about "power over" but "power to." If power is conceived as "power to," then students and teachers are both empowered by the liberating force of co-learnership.

Curriculum as Teacher-Student Interactions or Dialogue

The most common agreement seems to be that curriculum is what actually occurs between and among persons in the educational enterprise and not some "plan" for learning that is reflected in written materials. Diekelmann (1988) states in her Dialogue and Meaning model that "curriculum is a dialogue among teachers, practitioners, and students on what will constitute the knowledge in the nursing curriculum and what role experience will play in the curriculum" (p. 144). She goes on to say that "dialogue is a joint reflection on a phenomenon; it is a deepening of experience for all participants; it is talking, generating questions, and possibly interpreting" (p. 145). Moccia (1988) asserts that "it is time for us to turn back to the swamp of interpersonal relations between student and teacher. It is time to focus on the process of education – the student-teacher relationship – rather than on its content or anything else" (p. 59). In this same article she states: "It is the authentic dialogue between people that makes any activity worthwhile, regardless of whether or not it is called successful by others" (p. 60).

Watson (1988), in addressing the University of Colorado proposed nurse doctorate program, stated that the change must "acknowledge faculty development needs for new teaching-learning methods and student-teacher interactive practices, e.g., shift from oppressive interactions to liberating interactions (or from maintenance learning to anticipatory-participatory learning) or emphasize faculty's role as expert learners rather than expert givers of information" (p. 4). Munhall (1988), in what she labels "Implications for Curriculum Within the Theme of the Aquarian Conspiracy," lists fostering community and searching for meaning, self-discovery, freedom, choices, and relationships as suggested processes. The implication here is that these processes are essential to the curriculum revolution. Bevis (1988) goes so far as to define curriculum as those transactions and interactions that take place between and among students and teachers with the intent that learning take place. She refers to Huebner's (1966) "opportunities for engagement" and believes that such opportunities are the material from which curriculum is made. She also states that "any mode of conceptualizing the nursing teacher's role in an authoritarian, frontal teaching, information-giving, control-laden way (ultimately politically oppressive) is antithetical to the caring paradigm that is nursing's moral imperative and nursing education's moral activity (which must be ultimately politically liberating)" (p. 22).

It seems, therefore, that a very high priority criterion is that the essence of curriculum rests in the quality of interactions between and among students and faculty. Professional educational programs rely on a changed relationship between teachers and students where the teacher's role is one of meta-strategist who raises questions and issues and dialogues with students so that they become partners in education, not objects of education.

Curriculum That Stresses Syntactical Learning

A second criterion revolves around what students think about. The present paradigm for education is content laden, so content laden, in fact, that students have little time to think. Bevis (1988) writes:

> *The mind is an awesomely powerful instrument. It can evoke memories that are as real and alive and full of feeling as the day of their occurrence. It can enact plans that are years in the making and complex in their execution. It can yearn, dream, imagine, envision, expunge, and intuit. It can follow a trail of clues so thin that there is hardly a smell of reality and leap through a chain of logic confounding in its convolutions. Its only limits are our inadequacy in its use, our unskilled handling of its superb potential, our waste of its vast abilities, our lack of vision of its limitless powers.*

In classes, we teachers reduce it to its most elementary functions: absorption, memorization, and recitation. We give lectures on the mistaken assumption that if the students don't hear us say it, they will not learn it. We assume further that lecture is the most effective and efficient way to teach. Lecture is oppressive and in most cases inadequate (p. 20). (Though I will go on record as believing lecture is a good tool for a limited number of things, it would be tangential to elaborate here.)

Therefore, a second criterion for our revolution's success would be that faculty use teaching methodologies that stress syntactical learning, which is characterized by viewing wholes, having insights and finding meanings, evaluating and projecting, and predicting from knowns to unknowns using both data and intuition. This type of learning enables people to make intuitive leaps and to trust them. It involves welding together theory and practice into praxis and helping students find practice-grounded patterns, examples, and models that support formation of personal general guides and paradigms and provide help in knowing when and under what circumstances one departs from these.

Curriculum as Critical and Creative Thinking

Most authors of the curriculum revolution have syntactical learning, as described above, as a major focus of education for nurses. This primarily involves critical and creative thinking, the search for meanings. Diekelmann (1988), in speaking of strategies that can be used in the new curricula, addresses the link between language and thinking and believes that "helping students understand the critical processes clinicians and teachers bring to nursing will help them understand the nature of critical thinking in nursing practice" (p. 151). Obviously, the critical thinking I am referring to is not as it is usually perceived – i.e., orderly, logical, objective, and scientific – but as grounded in subjective experience that, as Carolyn Oiler Boyd says, "scorn definition, procedure, determination, and abstractions" (1988, p. 66).

The criterion that arises from this rumination is regarding what students think about. The content-backed curriculum must be deflated, slimmed down and unpacked. Content has continually been added to the curriculum but seldom deleted. Students are graduated tired, overworked, burned out, and undereducated. As aftermath of the revolution, there must be an emphasis on content as the vehicle for learning, not the driver and dictator of timing, methodology, interactions, and evaluation. In other words, the new paradigms, rather than content burdened, will be interactive and educational process centered and oriented toward creative and critical thinking.

Reality-Based Learning: Being-in-the-World

Currently, curriculum is faith teaching. Teachers focus on content emanating from a string of questionable logic that dictates it be derived from philosophy, conceptual frameworks, and program, level, and course objectives. The selected content, which is usually what faculty think is discipline sanctioned, is taught on the faith that students will need that chosen bit of information at some time in their careers.

This must change. To be successful, the curriculum revolution must be both effective in enabling faculties to derive content differently and successful in grounding the student learning experiences in reality. Boyd (1988), in speaking about phenomenology as a foundation for curriculum says: "lived experience is the focus of attention in phenomenology. Experience is not what we think, but what we live through. It is existing in a world; and, in the phenomenological sense, communicates the indivisible experiencing subject and experienced object" (p. 69). Diekelmann approaches content or knowledge as both theoretical and practical. Regarding experience in nursing education, she maintains that it is "restructured from one of a place in which theory is matched or applied in a laboratory or clinical setting to one of being-in-the-world with patients and nurses through language" (1987, p. 3).

Tanner (1988) concludes her article "Curriculum Revolution: The Practice Mandate" by commenting:

> *I do not think of developing more elegant and detailed formal models to be passed on to the next generation of nurses, for them to take and apply in their practice. Rather, I am struggling with ways in which the concerns of practice can truly be addressed by our educational activities, where classroom learning might be the application of practice rather than the other way around (p. 214).*

Benner (1984) believes that expert clinical teachers can best teach through presenting paradigm cases. She says that these paradigm cases transmit more than can be conveyed through abstract principles or guidelines. She states, "in order for students to learn from another person's paradigm case, they must actively rehearse or imagine the situation. Simulations can be even more effective because they require action and decisions from the learner." (p. 9).

What emerges in most of my colleagues' writings is a concern for relevance, reality, and practice, so that not only does theory inform practice, but practice informs theory. There also emerges a commitment to content in nursing having a clinical base – a contextual reality. Students in such a model are not whisked around from clinical experience to clinical experience and bent and molded in an effort to correlate some ideal of "theory" to some ideal of "practice." Instead, theory and practice coalesce or merge in ways that are meaningful for grounding content so that the contextual rules have an opportunity to be tested in reality and surface as grist for dialogue and teacher-student and student-student interactions, thereby finding their acontextual component in developing experience/expertise.

Practicum Experiences

One tradition-defying statement by Benner (1984, p. 185) goes upstream against institutionalized policy. Approval and accrediting bodies positively forbid specialization at undergraduate levels. This injunction seems to have no basis in research. Benner suggests, based upon her research that "early clinical specialization in one area might be extremely advantageous in that it would give students an opportunity to learn about the process of acquiring advanced clinical knowledge." What Benner may be counseling here has more to do with remaining in one clinical setting long enough to acquire a repository of paradigm experiences in order to learn the processes whereby one develops expertise than with undergraduate specialization as such. I believe that not only are we mistaken about the need for students to experience all major nursing specialty settings, but it is detrimental to developing the clinical scholars we all desire.

Diekelmann (1988, p. 147) opposes the popular conception that classroom and clinical practice should be closely correlated. She states: "The objective of developing clinical expertise in students does not depend on a corresponding relationship between classroom and clinical instruction." Further to confound the traditionalist, Diekelmann continues: "Students need not have at least one experience in each specialty area, nor are particular specialty areas or experiences mandatory" (p. 148). She believes, as I do, that these choices are for students to make in collaboration with teachers and clinical specialists. If we do not treat students as co-equals in the educational process and dialogue with them about their options and the wisdom of their choices, how can we ever hope to graduate autonomous nurses? Our fifth criterion, then, would be that in the new era, clinical experiences will be chosen by students after dialogue with teachers, fellow students, and clinicians, according to where they may best obtain the experiences they need in order to learn what they need to learn.

The sixth criterion addresses the idea that flexibility, not rigidity, must be the rule. Individuality of student choices and needs will be in evidence so that not all students will be required to have the same or nearly the same learning experiences. Students might, if they like, pursue some clinical interest that will enable them to learn how to develop expertise.

Phenomenological Teaching Approaches

In new models, clinical practice realities become the modality for study and the approach is qualitative in methodology rather than quantitative. Phenomenology, hermeneutical analysis, poetics, and other qualitative methods form the teaching-learning modalities. Both Munhall (1988) and Watson (1985) speak of the phenomenological thrust of the "new" nursing. Watson, in speaking of the transpersonal caring relationship of the nurse, states:

> Human care can begin when the nurse enters into the life space or phenomenal field of another person, is able to detect the other person's condition of being (spirit, soul), feels this condition within him or herself, and responds to the condition in such a way that the recipient has a release of subjective feelings and thoughts he or she had been longing to release. As such, there is an intersubjective flow between the nurse and patient (p. 63).

Munhall states that "the social humandate for change calls us to conspire together in the transformation of behavioristic, externally driven curriculum to one that focuses on expanding consciousness and the subjective and inter-subjective experiences of being human" (p. 228). Boyd, in her paper "Phenomenology of Nursing," says:

> We stand vulnerably in the wake of a spiraling system of controls on human irregularity made possible by scientific progress. For some of us, the human condition what it means to exist, to be alive in a world seized by technology is an appropriate, even important focus for nursing. Existentialism and phenomenology provide a lens (1988, p. 66).

There is little doubt for me that both existentialism and phenomenology are the lenses through which our curricula will reach the goals of excellence in professional service. In essence, they give us intentionality, and they ground the curriculum in "being-in-the-world." In addition, unlike the scientific, they give us flexibility – the justification for looking at unconcealing, at coming to know, and at exploring together. These ideas are antithetical to the common scientific positions of right and wrong answers, categorization of humans, human predictability, and division into parts. These two modes, existentialism and phenomenology, express wholes and explore consciousness. In speaking of phenomenological themes and concepts, Boyd (1988) states

> These themes provide an open framework descriptive of the nature of being human: the first distinguishing feature of the phenomenological perspective. Rather than starting with a philosophy and constructing a curriculum, phenomenology grounds us only in an understanding of the nature of being human. There are fewer linear, derived guidelines and prescriptives, more openness, and more constancy in processes of choice (p. 67).

Benner, another of the leaders in the phenomenological movement in nursing, offers guidance for phenomenological teaching approaches. If one defines curriculum as teacher-student interactions, these methods become the essence of the revolution. Benner makes the case that "the proficient clinician compares past whole situations with current whole situations" (1984, p. 9). Wholeness is something the behaviorist-empiricist paradigms seldom examine. Further, she believes that paradigm cases can be used as case studies and can be taken up as paradigms by learners. She states, "simulations [using paradigm cases] provide the learner with opportunities to gain paradigm cases in a guided way."

Another phenomenological methodology, poetics, can be useful in teaching. Poetics is a natural outcome of phenomenology. Watson (1985, p. 92) addresses this when she characterizes poetizing as the "true vocation of the experiential phenomenologist." She builds her position on Levin (1983) and maintains that poetizing is "necessary in that transcendental depth phenomenology, if focused and reflective of depth human experiences, cannot be other than poetic." If our teaching is centered on helping students find meaning, then poetics is a necessary element. Watson goes on to say, "Poetic expression has the power to touch and move us, to open and transport us. Thus, the poetic quality is related to the experiential meaning and, indeed, deepens the meaning, the felt senses, so that there is increased openness to describe and preserve the truth and depth of the experience." Phenomenology is grounded in reality, in wholes, in reflection, in insight, in everyday events. Such, too, is hermeneutics. Hermeneutic inquiry examines the textual or language-semantic structure of everyday practical activity. It begins in the everyday practical roles and functions of nursing – what nurses actually do. Using hermeneutics, teachers and students seek meaning through language about practice. Diekelmann, Benner, Allen, and Tanner are among those whose writings support hermeneutics as a nursing educational mode.

Therefore, the seventh criterion reads: Clinical and classroom learning methodologies are qualitative rather than quantitative. Phenomenology, hermeneutical analysis, poetics, and other qualitative methods based upon humanistic-existentialism form the teaching-learning modalities.

Caring as the Moral Imperative of Nursing Education

Another striking common element among the leaders of this revolution is the emphasis on caring. Fifteen years ago caring was a *persona non grata* in nursing. It implied sentimentality and a gushy, valentine approach to nursing. A few mavericks, Leininger, Murray, Bevis, Watson, Ray, Glittenberg, Gardner, Gaut, Parse, Boyle, and Uhl, were puttering along, outside the mainstream, researching, writing, and speaking about caring. These pioneers all believed that caring was the central core of nursing and formed its moral structure. Since that time, research and writing about caring fill volumes and have revealed much about the nature of caring and its role in nursing and nursing education. Commitment to the centrality of caring to the curriculum revolution is evident in the work of Watson, Benner, Diekelmann, Bevis, and Munhall. Actually, if a vote were taken, I think most nurses would agree that caring holds and must continue to hold a dominant role in our philosophy, our research, and our practice. Therefore, it must pervade our curriculum.

Watson (1985) has put it very powerfully: "Caring is the moral ideal of nursing" (p. 29). That must be our driver, our monitor, our guide in curriculum matters. She goes on to say that the ends of caring are protection, enhancement, and preservation of human dignity. Her belief is capsulized in her statement that: "Nursing as a human science and human care is always threatened and fragile. Because human care and caring requires a personal, social, moral, and spiritual engagement of the nurse and a commitment to oneself and other humans, nursing offers the promise of human preservation in society." This is not hyperbole. In a world that is increasingly computer-driven, machine-operated and controlled, mechanistic, and scientific, a world where even our elementary and high schools are "competency" based (i.e., behavioristic), nursing may well be the sanctuary of those most capable of preserving, sustaining, and protecting our collective and individual humanity. Munhall (1988, p. 227) in effect supports this position when she says that "the language of caring, which has been confined to the private domain and largely to women, emerges now as an ethical principle grounded in the concept of social responsibility and the credo of nonviolence."

Caring is powerful. Benner (1984, p. 208) identified six qualities of power associated with the caring provided by nurses. These are transformative, integrative, advocacy, healing, participative/affirmative, and problem solving. Bevis (1982) says, "The process of caring is as central to nursing as problem solving or communicating. It is implied every time 'nursing care' is referred to. Instead of nursing care the emphasis is on nurse *caring*" (p. 127). Bevis identified caring as essential content in nursing curricula. She included the research by Murray and Bevis done in the 1970s on the nature of the caring process in a chapter in her curriculum book. Bevis (1988) pointed out that one of the primary responsibilities of teachers in the new curriculum is to nurture the caring role. Diekelmann agrees, stating that, "The focus of the curriculum is the struggle to understand nursing knowledge and nursing practice. Caring, as an ontologic state, is fundamental to the curriculum" (1988, p. 144).

Therefore the eighth criterion is caring, as the moral ideal of nursing pervades the curriculum and forms its ethical imperative. It is the philosophical, research, and practice embodiment of nursing's essence and the source of nursing power. It is reflected in nursing's response to society's needs and its commitment to humanitarian service. Without caring, nursing is not a humanistic professional service, but a series of mechanistic tasks.

Criteria Based on Common Sense

There are several criteria that arise not so much from agreement among leadership as from common sense. Some of these have received attention from voices of the revolution; some have received none. However, in the mainstream of higher education, the history of nursing as a unified discipline, and the direction of flow of the discipline's growth each provide some evidence regarding indicators of success.

Professional Education Is Based in the Arts and Humanities

In our search for legitimacy with our academic colleagues, nursing's movement from hospitals to academic settings was accompanied by a strong reliance upon empiricism and behaviorism. Nursing needed to be in control of its own practice, education, and research, and this required movement into settings of higher education. In addition, nurse educators thought that to be acceptable in these settings, they had to assume the shape and texture of scientific academicians. So our art, so treasured in hospital curricula, gave way to science, so treasured in college curricula.

As we have become more self-confident, we have relinquished our drive to be an "applied" science and developed our own unique science – human science. It is based upon an entirely different set of assumptions that match our mission and are holistic, humanistic, feminist, service-related, and ethical. These assumptions arise from a caring ethic, a humanities base, and an intersubjective reality of being-in-the-world. This is at the very heart of the paradigm shift that motivates our revolution.

Sakalys and Watson (1985) reviewed seven major studies of education done in the 1980s. From these reports, they drew commonalities in curricular recommendations. First among these was "restoration of the centrality of the liberal arts in elementary, secondary, post-secondary, and professional education." In other words, there was an overriding concern for liberal arts within all the major studies and reports done on higher education in the first half of the 1980s.

Watson (1988) cites as one of the essentials for this transition the fact that we "acknowledge the arts and humanities as essential for educated persons and caring professionals." Her proposal for the nurse doctorate at the University of Colorado has a "more extensive liberal arts foundation" as its first principle. One of Boyd's concluding recommendations in her "Phenomenology for Nursing" (1988) is, not surprisingly, to "expand the use of the humanities in the nursing process." I believe we have stressed the sciences at the expense of humanities too long in nursing. The tradition of Florence Nightingale is one of the liberally educated woman. Following this model, nurses would be classically educated prior to entering nursing. Today, instead of a classical education, we usually require two to four courses in chemistry, two in anatomy and physiology, two in psychology (usually general introduction and pathology), two in math (general algebra and statistics), and one each in growth and development, sociology, nutrition, microbiology, and occasionally physics. Students are usually allowed to choose one humanities course among speech, art appreciation, music appreciation, and philosophy. They are required to take some literature, and this nod toward the great thoughts of human history is considered enough not only for nursing students but for most undergraduates in colleges and universities today.

Art, literature, poetry, music, philosophy, and architecture impart wisdom. They speak to that universal experience of humankind that unites and harmonizes. In the metaphors of art, poetry, music, and architecture, human suffering and transcending courage find their expression. Compassion and identification with the progress of human thought comes through literature and philosophy. Science may give us the tools for curing, but it is the humanities that give us the tools for caring. When we put a humanities base in nursing curriculum, we elevate nursing to its place in human concerns and empower it, as Watson (1985) says, truly to protect, enhance, and preserve human dignity. More than that, we as nurses can be persuasive in preserving humanness in the healing technological jungle.

Therefore, the ninth criterion is that the curriculum include courses in art, music, literature, and philosophy. In addition, nursing content should be approached using a humanities perspective.

Accessibility and Flexibility

The nudge toward accessibility and flexibility comes from the nature of the present world of students. Based on first-time candidates or the July 1988 NCLEX, associate degree programs now graduate 57 percent and diploma programs 10 percent of the total. This means that about 67 percent of new nurses lack the first professional degree. Increasing numbers of students no longer enter the profession immediately after high school; many are reentry persons with either second careers or second degrees, and more students than ever before work 20 or more hours per week. These realities force nurse educators to plan programs that allow ADN graduates to seek baccalaureate degrees with the least possible problems, roadblocks, and redundancy. It forces us to examine and to reconstruct our programs of study in such areas as the policies governing entry, part-time study, scheduling, articulation, and challenge exams or transfer of credit. We must arrange our programs so that they are flexible and accessible. Further, our courses and treatment of students must acknowledge that a large number of our students are adults with whom we should interact as adult to adult and in ways that enrich both the student and the teacher.

The tenth criterion is that policies, guidelines, and programs of study are formulated in ways that provide for flexibility and accessibility in order to respond to the needs of the associate degree and other nontraditional students. The eleventh is that course construction and teacher-student interactions are forged in ways that acknowledge the adult nature of the learner.

Noncurricular Indicators of Success

Curriculum is not the only thing that must change in order for the new era to arrive. Other conditions are necessary to success. Three that can be viewed with a sense of certainty that the curriculum revolution is accomplishing its goals are paradigm-free accreditation and approval criteria and procedures, faculty development and education in new age teaching modalities, and alteration in the health care practice environments.

Paradigm-Free Accreditation and Approval Criteria

It is almost embarrassing to say the obvious, but to omit it would be presumptuous. All these ideals of the revolution are of no use unless we are able to alter the criteria for national accreditation and state approval so that we can have indicators of excellence rather than paradigm-related criteria. Almost all state boards of nursing have, not in their nurse practice acts but in their rules and regulations governing educational programs, criteria that require that the products of the Tylerian/behavioristic/technological model be explicit in the curriculum-planning documents.

The National League for Nursing criteria for accrediting programs are also paradigm related. Though these criteria have, in the last two editions, eased up somewhat from the rigidity of the behaviorist paradigm, they have not altered in the *de facto* criteria.

The *de facto* criteria are those that, in fact, are used by the site visitors in their efforts to verify, clarify, and amplify. The *de facto* criteria are also used by state boards of review in determining the merit of programs. These criteria still tend to be strongly behaviorist-paradigm related. This may be due to such factors as:

1. The orientation of visitors and new board members
2. The pairing of experienced visitors with new ones so that socialization into the process overrides orientation and real criteria
3. The staggering of board membership so that an entirely new board is not possible, therefore old traditions die hard
4. The explanatory materials for accreditation criteria that may enhance the idea that paradigm-related criteria are still very much in force

These paradigm-required products of curriculum development that are so revered by state approval and national accreditation requirements are: a philosophy, conceptual framework, or at least concepts and threads; measurable/behavioral objectives for program, level, course, and units; a required program of study; clearly outlined content that accomplishes the objectives; and evaluation strategies that measure students' ability to meet the required behaviors specified in the objectives. It is clear that there are inherent obstacles in nursing that prevent any changes in paradigm. Until this is altered, all of our revolution is rhetoric, for no one will jeopardize state approval even if he or she is willing to forego national accreditation...

Therefore, the fourteenth indicator of success is the establishment of criteria for state approval and national accreditation of schools of nursing that stress research-based indicators of good schools of nursing and are paradigm-free.

Faculty Preparation and Development

There is a popular belief that graduate level nursing programs should no longer offer functional specialization on either the master's or the doctoral level. The belief is based upon the assumption that teaching nursing is not unique, and therefore if nursing teachers are interested in education courses, they should take them in schools of education. These same people believe that only clinical specialization is appropriate at the master's level. They also believe that if teachers are clinical specialists, productive researchers, and published, they are *ipso facto* good teachers.

One of the earmarks of a profession is that is has sanctioned ways to educate for the profession. Nursing has certainly illustrated that, with its institutionalization of the Tyler/behaviorist paradigm. However, anyone who has taken courses in schools of education knows that these courses are primarily geared to elementary and secondary school levels, are based upon non-practice field norms, and have little relevance for classroom and clinical teaching for nursing. Just having intelligence enough to make some transfer from those levels is not enough. So much of what is said is inappropriate to the practice field of nursing and so much of what is appropriate and needed is not said or known. In fact, so much of what we now teach in nursing education courses does not help teachers struggle with helping students learn things that nurses must learn in order to serve society. These nontangible necessities include finding meanings, using intuition safely, examining assumptions, gaining insights, seeing patterns, recognizing significance and implications, being caring and concerned, being idealistic, making moral and ethical commitments, building a background of paradigm experiences, identifying as a professional nurse, inquiring into the nature of things, being creative, strategizing, thinking critically, and knowing about power, its use, control, and limits. Whatever teacher education we have must help teachers learn to teach these things. My concept of the new age curriculum development paradigms rests upon an altered role of the teacher – one in which the teacher is an expert nurse and an expert learner who knows how to help others become expert nurses and learners.

Further, we have long accepted the fact that health care agencies must have staff development departments with full-time persons employed as teachers of the staff. As educators, we have assumed that we do not need this and that the occasional workshop or meeting suffices to keep us up to date. That time must pass. Faculty must consistently have access to a colleague-teacher who helps plan and furnish an organized and orderly curriculum in both nursing and educational content so that faculty stay on the cutting edge of expertise and knowledge. In turn, faculty need to have a trusted colleague who helps them change or maintain the roles of teaching through simulation, inquiry, and dialogue.

These ideas lead us to two criteria for success of the revolution: graduate schools on the master's and/or doctoral level offer courses in nursing education with an emphasis on both clinical expertise and educative teaching skills; and faculties employ full-time faculty/staff development personnel to enable educators to maintain their clinical and teaching expertise.

Alienation in the Health Care System

If the revolution is a success, and I believe it will be, the graduates of professional programs will have characteristics of professionals, meaning that they will be creative, critical thinkers, ethically astute, professionally autonomous, independent, and collegial in their relationships. These characteristics do not make for good institutional employees. Hospitals are showing the strain of too few nurses and too many slots to fill. Nursing seems to be taking the brunt of the criticism for not graduating enough students. This is not a nursing problem; it is an industry problem.

One of the most severe problems of the industry is that it has become a mega-bureaucracy with more of an eye for profits than for people. Nurses traditionally are of the proletariat and identify with the people. They see large numbers of the population without health care coverage, they see creaking and straining in the system from cost to insurers and government, and they see themselves treated as employees without privileges instead of knowledgeable professionals.

Due to the shifts in the health care scene that I mentioned at the beginning of the chapter, there are increasing numbers of people being cared for in the home. Somewhere I have heard that home health care is the fastest growing industry in the United States and I have no reason to doubt it, though I cannot document it. One solution is that professional nurses move out of hospitals into home health, where they traditionally have more room for creativity and autonomy. Yet, we cannot abandon those who are the most ill, the most vulnerable, the least able to care for themselves, and the most needy. Professional nurses must remain in hospitals as well as move to home health agencies and nursing homes. To do that we must make health care agencies more hospitable to professional nurses. Now is the time; times of acute shortages are times of change. Now is the time to commence massive negotiations with hospitals, nursing homes, and home health agencies for basic shifts in their attitudes and policies about nurses and to enlist their aid in altering educational practices and state nursing acts regarding the constraints on both education and practice.

My fifteenth and last criterion for success of the paradigm shift in nursing education is that practice settings must change so that they are hospitable places for nurses to exercise the new ways of being that are characteristic of the substantively different professional graduates of the new curricula.

Conclusion

These criteria (Figure 1) are rough, but for the most part they hit at the heart of the revolution. They point toward the significant and substantive changes that must occur if this revolution is to succeed. I would like them used as a working paper, to be altered and refined and ultimately used to help map the revolution.

Figure 1: Paradigm Changes

First Principle:

Any and all changes in paradigm must in some way affect the liberation and empowerment of people – both students and teachers.

Criteria:

1. Professional educational programs rely on a changed relationship between teachers and students, wherein the teacher's role is one of meta-strategist who raises questions and issues and dialogues with students so that they become partners in education, not objects of education.

2. Faculty use teaching methodologies that stress syntactical learning, which is characterized by viewing wholes, having insights, seeing patterns, finding meanings, evaluating, and predicting using both data and intuition.

3. Curriculum is interaction and educational process centered, oriented toward creative and critical thinking and not content burdened.

4. Clinical practice realities are the foci of study so that content in nursing has a contextual reality.

5. Clinical experiences are chosen by students after dialogue with teachers, fellow students, and clinicians, according to where they may best obtain the experiences they need.

6. Students need not all have similar learning experiences. Students may pursue some clinical interests that will enable them to learn how to develop expertise.

7. Phenomenology, hermeneutical analysis, poetics, and other qualitative methods based upon humanistic existentialism form the teaching-learning modalities.

8. Caring, as the moral ideal of nursing, pervades the curriculum and forms its ethical imperative. It is the philosophical, research, and practice embodiment of nursing's essence and the source of nursing power. It is reflected in nursing's response to society's needs and its commitment to humanitarian service.

9. The curriculum includes courses in art, music, literature, and philosophy. In addition, nursing content is approached using a humanities perspective.

10. Policies, guidelines, and programs of study are formulated in ways that provide for flexibility and accessibility in order to respond to the needs of the nontraditional student.

11. Course construction and teacher-student interactions are forged in ways that acknowledge the adult nature of the learner.

12. Graduate schools on the master's and/or doctoral level offer courses in nursing education with an emphasis on both clinical expertise and educative teaching skills.

13. Faculties' developmental needs are met by employing full-time faculty/staff development personnel to enable faculty to maintain their clinical and teaching expertise.

14. National accreditation and state-approval mechanisms rest on research-based indicators of excellence that are not related to a curriculum paradigm.

15. Practice settings must change so that they are hospitable places for nurses to exercise the new ways of being that are characteristic of the substantively different professional graduates of the new curricula.

We cannot only meet, talk, and write papers; we must organize for change. The National League for Nursing has already formed an informal central planning group whose mission is to establish goals for the revolution. This group, or another similar group, needs to form task forces, each assigned to a separate criterion. These task forces must then plan and execute a national effort to attack the problems and issues relevant to meeting the criteria. Without such an effort our revolution will be slipshod, bloody, self-destructive to nursing, without rigor, and unresponsive to society's needs. We must form a coalition in common cause to improve nursing on behalf of the people we serve.

I end with this thought:

> There is a compelling splendor about both teaching and nursing that demand the highest forms of endeavor, for their ends are linked to the magnificent miracle of human thought and the quality of human life. They have a common core of caring about the human condition and an obligation to its improvement that confers a radiant beauty on the meanest of tasks in their service. They are a societal trust. And, for those who combine these two tasks into the teaching of nursing, there is a moral commitment to society s needs that requires industrious constancy in improving care so that this trust will be steadfastly and excellently honored. It is to this trust that our revolution is dedicated. (Bevis, 1988, p. 1)

References

Benner, P. (1984). *From novice to expert: Excellence and power in clinical nursing practice.* Menlo Park, CA: Addison-Wesley.

Bevis, E. (1982). *Curriculum building in nursing: A process.* St. Louis, MO: Mosby.

Bevis, E. (1988). Teacher as educator: Some directions for faculty development. In E. Bevis & J. Watson (Eds.), *A new direction for curriculum development for professional nursing: A paradigm shift From training to education.* Unpublished manuscript.

Boyd, C. O. (1988). Phenomenology: A foundation for nursing curriculum. In *Curriculum revolution: Mandate for change* (pp. 65-87). New York: National League for Nursing.

Diekelmann, N. L. (1987). *Alternate models for professional nursing education: New approaches for nursing curriculum development.* Unpublished manuscript.

Diekelmann, N. L. (1988). Curriculum revolution: A theoretical and philosophical mandate for change. In *Curriculum revolution: Mandate for change* (pp. 137-157). New York: National League for Nursing.

Felton, G. M., & Parsons, M A. (1984). *The effect of education on the ability to resolve ethical/moral dilemmas.* Unpublished manuscript.

Huebner, D. (1966). Curriculum language and classroom meanings. In J. Macdonald & R. Leeper, (Eds.), *Language and meaning*. Washington, DC: Association for Supervision and Curriculum Development.

Levin, D. (1983). The poetic function in phenomenological discourse. In W. McBride & C. Schrag (Eds.), *Phenomenology in a pluralistic context*. Albany, NY: State University of New York Press.

Moccia, P. (1988). Curriculum revolution: An agenda for change. In *Curriculum revolution: Mandate for change* (pp. 53-64). New York: National League for Nursing.

Munhall, P. (1988). Curriculum revolution: A social mandate for change. In *Curriculum revolution: Mandate for change* (pp. 217-230). New York: National League for Nursing.

Rest, J. (1979). *Manual for the defining issues test: An objective test of moral judgment* (rev. ed.). Minneapolis: University of Minnesota.

Sakalys, J., & Watson, J. (1985). New directions in higher education: A review of trends. *Journal of Professional Nursing, 1*(5), 293-299.

Tanner, C. A. (1988). Curriculum revolution: The practice mandate. In *Curriculum revolution: Mandate for change* (pp. 201-216). New York: National League for Nursing.

Watson, J. (1985). *Nursing: Human science and human care: A theory of nursing*. Norwalk, CT: Appleton- Century-Crofts.

Watson, J. (1988). Curriculum in transition. In *Curriculum revolution: Mandate for change* (pp. 1-8). New York: National League for Nursing.

Curriculum Revolution: The Practice Mandate[1]

Christine A. Tanner

Embedded in our everyday lives are worldviews and beliefs about the self that profoundly affect the way we live. Yet these remain largely implicit and unspoken. They can become apparent as we strive with others to interpret our spoken message and our actions. Understanding such implicit assumptions can also be emancipatory. To that end, this chapter will make explicit some of the views and assumptions that have been embedded in and have dominated our practice as nurse educators.

The first part of the chapter is drawn largely from the writing of Donald Schon, an MIT (Massachusetts Institute of Technology) social scientist who has done a thoughtful study of the practice professions and their place in higher education (Schon, 1983). This is primarily to provide some context for the second and more important part of the chapter. In part 2, I will explore the way in which we have formalized the concerns of practice in our nursing curricula, focusing on long-standing assumptions about the nature of nursing practice, in general, and about the nature of clinical judgment in nursing, in particular.

The Technical Rationality Model of Knowledge

Schon (1983) claims that the model of what he terms technical rationality has dominated the education of professions. In this view, professional activity consists of "instrumental problem solving made rigorous by application of scientific theory and technique" (p. 21). Practice consists of problem solving based on specialized scientific knowledge. The work of the professional is to be thoroughly familiar with knowledge that has been developed and tested through research, and then apply this knowledge to solving the problems of everyday practice. This view of practice and the relationship between knowledge and practice has powerfully shaped our thinking in nursing education.

At first it may be difficult to consider the possibility that there exists another viable point of view; that is, that professional practice should or could consist of other than rational problem solving founded on a sound scientific base. This is, after all, the dominant view of nursing practice. It shows up everywhere in the literature on the relationship between theory, practice, and research. Common views about this relationship are: (1) theory and research exist to guide our practice; (2) the best practice is research-based; and (3) there is a need for more systematic research by which to provide a scientific basis for our practice. Although many authors acknowledge that questions for research might derive from practice, the flow of knowledge is clearly from research and theory to practice. The clinician is often faulted

1.Originally published in *Curriculum revolution: Mandate for change*
(1988, pp. 201-216). New York: National League for Nursing.
Reprinted with permission.

because of his or her failure to use research in practice. As a result, large-scale projects have been mounted to promote clinicians' use of research.

Schon (1983) points out that this notion of application leads to a view of professional knowledge as a hierarchy in which general principles occupy the highest level and concrete problems occupy the lowest. According to Schein (1973), there are three components to professional knowledge: (1) an underlying discipline, or basic science component, upon which practice rests or from which it is developed; (2) an applied science component from which many day-to-day diagnostic procedures and problem solutions are derived; and (3) a skills and attitudinal component concerning the actual performance of services to the client, using the underlying basic and applied knowledge.

In nursing, we order our curricula along the same lines of this hierarchy. First we study the basic sciences as foundational to the applied science of nursing. For example, we assume that we cannot study asepsis until the course in microbiology is completed. Hand washing is the skill component for our applied study of asepsis. As an aside, let me point out that this hierarchy of knowledge is paralleled in the hierarchy of nursing roles. The scientist has highly esteemed status, then educators who help apply the science, and finally the clinicians at the bottom of the hierarchy.

The assumptions embedded in our curricular practices are not unlike those of other professions. But it is time to examine the assumptions that practice is only rigorous problem solving when applying scientific principles, and that the important and true knowledge for practice is derived from scientific research.

Schon (1983) claims that there is a crisis in the practice disciplines because this view of knowledge for practice does not meet the reality of practice. He describes the changing character of situations in practice that limit the utility of traditional scientific knowledge as the primary route to problem resolution. He points out several characteristics of practice: complexity, instability, uncertainty, and value conflict. Let us examine these characteristics more closely as they pertain to the practice of nursing, then reflect on the potential for a usable, standardized, and generalizable knowledge base for practice.

Complexity

Our scientific knowledge specifies that, all things being equal, a certain percentage of patients will respond positively to a particular intervention. Seldom in practice are all things equal. Moreover, we seldom know the extent to which this patient is like the greater proportion of patients who responded positively to the intervention. The judgment to use a scientifically based intervention is far more complex than what is assumed by the model of technical rationality and the instrumental application of scientifically based knowledge.

Instability

Our practice is changing rapidly and the development of scientific knowledge is hardly keeping pace. Because of this, too many questions in practice remain unanswered. Even if professional knowledge were to catch up with the new demands of practice, the improvement in professional performance would be transitory. The role of the nurse will continually be reshaped over the next decades by the reorganization of health and disease care. As the role changes, so will the demand for usable knowledge.

Uncertainty

The situations of practice are not problems to be solved but are problematic situations characterized by uncertainty, ambiguity, and indeterminacy. Nurses are not confronted with problems that are independent of one another but with dynamic situations of inordinate complexity and changing, interacting problems. Schon (1983) cites Russell Ackoff, who refers to such situations as "messes." Problems are abstractions extracted from "messes" by analysis.

Value Conflicts

Practitioners are frequently embroiled in conflicts of values, goals, purposes, and interests. Nurses are faced with pressures for increased efficiency in the context of contracting budgets. Patients are sent home without an adequate system of care; the goals of the institution for containing costs may be in direct conflict with the goals of quality patient care.

In summary, the argument Schon (1983) offers is based on four aspects: (1) that practice has traditionally been viewed as the instrumental application of research-based knowledge to problem solving; (2) that our educational approaches reflect a hierarchy with practice knowledge derived from higher forms of knowledge; (3) that the higher up in the hierarchy of knowledge, the more standardized and generalizable it is; and (4) that the kinds of problems (or "messes") faced by nurses in their practice requires far greater knowledge than that which is offered by traditional science. Schon offers a serious challenge to the way in which we think about practice, and the way in which we organize our curricula as a reflection of this view. An alternative conception of knowledge and the relationship between knowledge and practice may be instructive to our deliberations about curriculum change.

Other Views of Knowledge and Their Relationship to Practice

The notion that there are multiple ways of knowing may now be familiar through the writings of such scholars as Munhall (1982), Oiler (1982), Carper (1978), and Benner (1983, 1984; Benner & Wrubel, 1982). Benner has brought to nursing some very important notions about knowing drawn from Polanyi and the Heideggerian view of being in the world. In Benner's study of expert nurses, she found that nurses discover ways to deal competently with the ambiguities and value conflicts of practice.

There is a knowing in practice that shows up in the spontaneous, intuitive performance of the actions of everyday life. This knowing, in Polanyi's (1958) terms, is tacit, implicit in our patterns of action and in our feel for the stuff with which we are dealing. It seems that this knowing is embedded in the practice. Every competent practitioner can recognize phenomena, a pattern associated with a way of coping, or more subtle patterns that serve as an early warning of an impending problem, for which the practitioner cannot give a reasonably accurate or complete description.

To provide an illustration of such tacit knowing, I refer to our study on intuition in clinical judgment (Benner & Tanner, 1987). We observed nurses in the intensive care unit, and interviewed them about their judgments. One nurse was caring for a young female patient who was suffering from a liver disease that sometimes affects pregnant women. The woman appeared unresponsive. In response to my opening question about the patient's status, the nurse stated:

> She s more responsive than she was yesterday, but it s not real consistent. Most of the time she ll open her eyes when you talk with her. She says she s not in any pain, but I find this hard to believe because she s had a C section. She s got that awful tube in her mouth, and we tie her down. She s more cooperative when we go to turn her, when we tell her whether we re turning her to her left or to her right. Then she starts swinging her body a little bit, not like lifting her arm up and going for the side rail, but not as resistant as she was yesterday.

This kind of qualitative distinction is difficult to describe. Yet this nurse was unusual in her ability to provide illustrations of her judgment concerning the slightly improved health of her patient. But difficulty in describing is not a case of being inarticulate. Rather, it is an implicit knowing that has not been formalized in rational language as appropriate scientific thought. In day-to-day practice, the nurse makes innumerable judgments of quality for which she cannot state adequate criteria or rules. And even when the clinician makes conscious use of research-based theories and techniques, he or she is dependent on tacit recognitions, judgments, and skillful performances.

Benner (1983), drawing on the work of Polanyi and Kuhn, has made a distinction between "knowing that" and "knowing how." "Knowing that" knowledge is the formal knowledge in the curriculum, the instrumental and theoretical knowledge that makes up the course taught in the classroom. "Knowing how," or tacit knowledge, is practical knowledge and dependent on experience. In our approach to curriculum development, we have recognized as legitimate only theoretical knowing, and have largely neglected the knowledge of experience.

The possibility that the technical model of higher education for the professions may not be the most functional in terms of preparing skilled clinicians is now apparent. However, there is an alternative model that, while accepting theoretical knowledge as a necessary ingredient for learning from practice, elevates the status of practice and knowledge from practice to being the lifeblood of expert performance. There is a knowing in practice that can and must inform our curriculum planning.

Formalization of Knowledge in the Curriculum

The curriculum is our best attempt to formalize the knowledge and skills needed for practice. It is our way to put into language the concern of practice as we understand it. By concern in practice, I mean the kinds of issues with which nurses must deal. For example, in practice, we are concerned with making the best clinical judgments possible; we must prepare nurses to make astute clinical judgments, to make accurate and relevant observations, to draw inferences from those observations, and to determine appropriate nursing actions. In our curricula, we have formalized this concern as a rational, sequential model of problem solving – the nursing process – frequently operationalized as the written nursing care plan.

In the 1960s, the formalization of the nursing process was a revolutionary development. It was an acknowledgment that nurses were thinkers, not just doers. It was the application of the scientific method applied to practice. But we must ask now, in the 1980s, does this formalization capture the essence of clinical judgment?

Before I consider this question in more detail, I will provide other illustrations of this way of thinking about curriculum, that is, that curriculum is the formalization of practice concerns. Illness, of course, is another concern in practice, the lived experience of our patients in coping with their diseases, their symptoms, and their changes in life style. The formalization of illness, however, quite often is disease, with the symptom being viewed as an indicator of the disease rather than an experience that has meaning for the patient. Another concern in practice is caring, our intimate connectedness with inordinate healing power. Its formalization is empathy, therapeutic communication, advocacy, and assertiveness. This interpretation of practice concerns and their formalization may not be met with unanimous agreement, but it does provide a vehicle to think about why we have included certain kinds of content in the curriculum and in what way that material may (or may not) be related to practice.

Now formalization is not an evil. A formalization is essential to provide the novice with guideposts and rules for safe entry into professional practice. However, formalizations have some characteristics that tell us that they must frequently and carefully be scrutinized for the adequacy with which they represent practice. These characteristics include the following:

1. A formalization is a representation. It gives us a way to view a situation. But it is only one representation and there may be other perspectives. It is not absolute truth.

2. As a representation and as one view, a formalization may miss the target.

3. Formalizations are inevitably incomplete.

4. The formalization may be so abstract that multiple meanings are possible (and even likely) and the intended meaning is lost. For example, the maxim that nursing treats the whole patient is quite abstract and there are multiple concrete interpretations of this maxim.

5. There is a profound tendency to deify our formalization as being identical to the concern. Then we lose sight of the original concern. Such is the case, I believe, with the nursing process as substitute for the practice concern of clinical judgment.

The Formalization and the Practice of Clinical Judgment

Let us now take a closer look at the concern in practice of clinical judgment and its formalization in the nursing process. In this section, I will discuss some of my own research on clinical judgment and some of the turns that it has taken as a result of my own new awareness.

As a beginning nurse educator in the early 1970s, I adopted the prevailing approach to teaching clinical judgment as the nursing process. It provided a clear step-by-step linear approach to nursing judgments, a rational model that encouraged the students to clearly identify their assessment data, their plans stated as patient-centered objectives, their nursing orders and the accompanying scientific rationale, and their evaluation of the effectiveness and efficiency of the plan. I gradually became aware of the fact that while some students could write elegant care plans, these same students lacked flexibility to respond to rapidly changing practice situations, or the practical know-how to truly do the interventions. What I was most keenly aware of was that these students had no sense of salience regarding assessment data. They would collect it, and this practice seemed to get no better with time. Moreover, they seemed to have no ability to extract any meaning from the data.

In 1975, I began to research clinical problem solving. In the 10 years that followed, in an effort to understand the underlying processes of clinical judgment, I applied a rational/cognitive model of problem solving to the study of nursing students and nurses. My implicit assumption, which I did not understand until just recently, was that clinical judgment is a rational process. The meaning of this will become clear through illustrations from the research.

Actually, there are several approaches to the study of clinical judgment within the rationalist paradigm. The typical study is directed at one of two goals: (1) to compare the performance of clinicians in deriving a decision with that prescribed by a statistical model or (2) to describe the actual thought processes used by clinicians in deriving a diagnosis or determining appropriate interventions.

As an example of the former, Grier (1976) conducted a study to determine if "intuitive" decisions by nurses were in agreement with those derived by a statistical model. The model used describes the selection of an action or set of actions based on a subjective assignment of value to probable outcomes of those actions. The use of this model requires the assignment of the likelihood of certain outcomes associated with specified actions. Each outcome also has some value assigned to it. Given these subjectively assigned probabilities and values, it is possible to derive mathematically the preferred outcome. It assumes that the human judge is an intuitive statistician, that it is preferable to quantify the probabilities and values, and that the resulting decision will be better than if these probabilities and values are left unspecified. It also assumes that we can specify all relevant attributes of the situation to feed into the model.

Grier (1976) compared the decisions made intuitively with those made by the mathematical model and found agreement nearly 60 percent of the time. She concluded that a systematic and objective process was used in making most of these decisions, resulting in a justifiable choice of action for achieving the desired goal.

In my own research, I rejected this model, since my interest was more in line with attempting to describe the actual thought processes of clinical judgment. My work, up until recently, was placed squarely on information processing theory drawn from the work of Newell and Simon (1972) in artificial intelligence. This theory describes problem solving behavior as an interaction between an information processing system (the problem solver) and a task environment (the task, as described by the experimenter). It is assumed that human information processing capacity is limited by memory constraints, and that strategies must be used to adapt these limitations to the demands of the task environment.

The model of diagnostic reasoning advanced by Elstein, Shulman, and Sprafka (1978) describes strategies that diagnosticians use to adapt to the large amounts of information available in most diagnostic tasks. The model includes four major activities: (1) problem sensing, attending to initially available cues; (2) activating diagnostic hypotheses that may explain the initial cues presented; (3) gathering data that generally are hypothesis-directed (i.e., data are sought for ruling in, ruling out, or refining the hypothesis); and (4) evaluating the hypotheses.

Elstein, et al argued that early hypotheses serve as a "chunking" mechanism, conserving short-term memory space by clustering clinical data into familiar diagnostic patterns. My associates and I sought to determine if this model of diagnostic reasoning described the strategies used by nurses and junior and senior nursing students (Tanner, Padrick, Westfall, & Putzier, 1987; Westfall, Tanner, Putzier, & Padrick, 1986). Subjects were presented with brief videotaped vignettes depicting a patient experiencing one or more problems. The subjects' task was to seek additional information from the examiner until they had derived the most likely diagnosis(es) and determined appropriate interventions. During their information seeking, they were instructed to "think aloud;" these verbalizations were transcribed and analyzed for the number and type of diagnostic hypotheses; the earliness with which hypotheses were activated; the number of cues sought in information gathering; the type of information-gathering approach (e.g., hypothesis testing, cue exploration); the adequacy of the information used to evaluate the diagnostic hypotheses; and the accuracy of the diagnosis. They found that all subjects activated diagnostic hypotheses early. Groups could be distinguished by only two measures: the degree to which they used systematic information gathering and the accuracy of the final diagnosis.

Several other studies on clinical judgment in nursing have been conducted within the rationalist perspective. Hammond, Kelly, Schneider, and Vancini (1967) conducted the only other study comparing nursing performance with a statistical model. Corcoran (1986a, 1986b) used information processing theory to study the processes used by expert and novice hospice nurses in making decisions regarding administration of pain medications. Other investigators (Gordon, 1980; Cianfrani, 1984; Matthews & Gaul, 1979) have used concept attainment theory as a framework for research on processes of nursing diagnosis.

A singular perception emerges from these studies within the rationalist perspective: the nursing process does not capture the dynamic interactive thinking processes of diagnosis or planning. The process clearly is not as linear as we might think. Those of us involved in this area of research are now questioning the extent to which the written nursing care plan, as the primary instructional method, is likely to be helpful to nursing students in learning this dynamic process (Tanner, 1987; Corcoran, 1986a).

Along with this insight from the research, the rational model also did not seem to capture some of the more important aspects of clinical judgment. There were numerous unexplained phenomena, such as the ability to zero in on the right region for assessment, the ability to recognize which data are important to attend to and which can be ignored, the ability to recognize a pattern and act on that recognition without consciously labeling it, and the important role of emotion in clinical judgment.

In contrast, the rational model (as emphasized in nursing process, information processing theory, decision theory, and the model of technical rationality previously described) assumes that action is the result of rational and logical procedures mediated by cognitive processes. When these are not obvious or do not show themselves in the protocols of experts, it is that the processes are too rapid to access. In other words, they are unconscious. The rational model also assumes it is possible to make explicit and to formalize the knowledge used by the clinician in making judgments.

About the time that these concerns regarding the research model were rising, Benner (1984) published her early work on the development of expertise in nursing. Her work, as well as that of others (Pyles & Stern, 1983; Phillips & Rempusheski, 1985), provides a stark contrast to the rationalist models. Benner's initial work, as well as subsequent research on the role of intuition in clinical judgment (Benner & Tanner, 1987), uses hermeneutic inquiry, based on Heideggerian phenomenology.

Hermeneutic Inquiry

The object of study in hermeneutic inquiry is the semantic or textual structure of everyday practical activity, what people actually do when they are engaged in the practical tasks of life. Heidegger (1962) distinguished three modes of engagement that people have with their surroundings. The *practical mode* is the most basic. This is the mode of practical day-to-day activities, in which one's awareness is essentially holistic; that is, persons' awareness of the situation in which they are engaged is not as an arrangement of discrete physical objects, but as a network of interrelated projects. The *reflective mode* is entered when the individual encounters some problem in practical activity. The source of the breakdown of action becomes salient in a way it was not in the ready-to-hand mode. The source of the breakdown is still seen as an aspect of the task, rather than as a context-free object. The *theoretic mode* is entered only when the individual detaches him or herself from ongoing practical activity and relies on the use of rational, logical processes to deal with the breakdown.

In this view, the practical mode characterizes expert clinical judgment. The expert's perspective of a patient situation is holistic, not broken down into discrete elements. This is contrary to the rationalist assumption that expert clinical judgment is characterized by detached theorizing and analytic logical processes.

The practical mode also is the starting place for hermeneutic inquiry. The study of clinical judgment using hermeneutics is the study of what nurses actually do when they are engaged in the practical tasks of delivering nursing care. The hermeneutic approach seeks to make explicit the practical understanding of human actions through their interpretation.

In her study of skill acquisition, Benner (1984) interviewed and observed experienced nurses, newly graduated nurses, and senior nursing students, as well as pairs of newly licensed nurses and their more experienced nurse preceptors. During the interviews, nurses were asked to describe situations that stood out for them. Using the interview and observation data for textual interpretation, Benner provided evidence that expert judgment derives from a grasp of the whole situation – a qualitative or perceptual assessment based on a combination of "the senses of touch, smell and sight and on the interpretation of a patient's physical, verbal and behavioral expression" (Benner & Wrubel, 1982, p. 12). These holistic judgments differed from the objective, measurable judgments such as those described in the rationalist models. In a study using grounded theory strategies, Pyles and Stern (1983) identified the formation of a "gestalt" or achievement of insight about a patient situation similar to Benner's description.

In subsequent research on clinical judgment within this perspective, Benner and Tanner (1987) described aspects of intuition. Drawing on the work of Dreyfus and Dreyfus (1986), they defined intuition as "understanding without a rationale" and not a "mystical or accidental human capacity" (p. 29). In their pilot study, expert nurses were interviewed and observed in their practice. The narrative accounts provided by the nurses contain rich descriptions of expert clinical judgment.

Several aspects of intuition described in this study are relevant to this discussion.

1. **Pattern recognition** is the perceptual ability that enables human beings to recognize configurations and relationships without analytically specifying the components of the patterns. A good example of this ability is face recognition; people do not analyze an individual's facial features, yet they are able to recognize people they have met by a memory of the overall facial "pattern." Patients present patterns that expert nurses learn to attend to. In contrast to this view of pattern recognition, rationalist models of clinical judgment treat pattern recognition either as a feature detection system, in which a list of features held in memory is matched against the features presented by the patient, or as a template matching scheme.

2. **Sense of salience** is the perception of things as being more or less important. The expert nurse, who has a sense of salience, will not consider all observations as pertinent; only some will stand out. Skilled observations of the patient over a long period of time allow the nurse to understand what is salient for this situation. A routine assessment checklist will not be as effective in situations that require highly individualized observations, such as the subtle changes occurring in head injured patients.

Now let us examine contrasting assumptions. In this view, action precedes analytic thought rather than occurring as a result of it. The knowing is in the doing, and we may theorize about it later. There are no formal strategies of clinical judgment that can be described free of the context in which the action occurs. Rather, an understanding of any human activity must be historically and contextually situated. The knowledge used as the basis for clinical judgment is practical, derived from experience with similar and dissimilar situations. The knowledge is embedded in the practice and may or may not be rendered explicit or formal. Rational, analytic approaches to clinical judgment are characteristic of beginner rather than expert performance.

What may we conclude from this regarding the formalization of clinical judgment as nursing process? It is a formalization that is ill-suited to expertise in practice. At best, it may serve as an introductory framework, which may quickly be abandoned as students gain some experience in their clinical work. It may also represent, somewhat inadequately, aspects of clinical judgment, but it cannot be considered the same as the processes of clinical judgment.

In my work with Benner, I had the opportunity to watch and talk with some of the best nurses I have ever seen. Their expertise in clinical judgment, their understanding of the lived experience of illness, their attitudes toward caring escaped the formalisms we currently use in our nursing programs. Finally, I would like to share with you an incredibly poignant paradigm case that captures the essence of this expertise and, at the same time, the limits of formalism. This paradigm case was presented by a skilled coronary care unit nurse during a group interview. The man she is discussing was in the coronary care unit for cardiomyopathy.

We had a young man, 22 years old, who I will never forget. He was about 2 and 1/2 hours from home, and up here by himself. I think he knew that he was very ill but he didn't really understand how ill. He didn't understand that he was actually terminal. The impression I had was that it was important for us as a nursing staff to know him as a person and to care for him. And he was very personable. I took care of him three days in a row for 12 hour shifts. I admitted him and chose to stay with him. He was very hopeful that something would be found, that he would feel better. Sometimes he would even say, "Oh, I don't feel too bad now." But his readings would be just about the same and really he didn't have an improvement. So he was really searching, I think, and it made my heart go out to him.

He made a point to share a lot of personal aspects of his life. And not everybody does that. [I: Give me an example of the kinds of things he shared.] What he liked to do with his free time, how he met his fiancé, how he never thought he would be in a hospital being so young, how he couldn't wait to go home because he had these things he planned to do, and the wedding was in 6 months and gee, he had never even been to a wedding before and now he was going to have his own. He told me what his fiancé did for a living, and how he hoped to go into business with his father. Things like that, little things but he seemed to want to talk about his life almost every time I went into his room. I don't know, maybe he did realize how sick he was.

[I: How did you respond to that?] It made me sad, but I was flattered that he wanted to talk to me. I just listened and would say, "Is that right?" or "How nice that you met this person." I didn't ask him, I wanted to let him say what he wanted to say.

They made the decision not to intubate him, even though it is a very hard decision to make, and you feel very ambivalent. He became very breathless. Now the point was just to make him as comfortable as possible. He felt more comfortable in the chair. So he sat in the chair. He wanted a popsicle. He got a popsicle. He wanted to drink some water. Fine, he could have water if he wanted it. We started giving him small doses of morphine to see if that would help with his anxiety. Medically, they didn't want to give more potent respiratory depressants like valium because they felt that that might harm him. However, in retrospect, I wish they could have calmed him somewhat. But it has given me tremendous empathy for people who are short of breath. It's an awful way to go because he was conscious to the very end. He also kept pulling me back. Anytime I tried to leave the room he would grab my arm and say, Don t leave me. Don t leave me. So I stayed with him and had someone else take over my other patient assignments.

I held his hand, I rubbed his neck. We brought a radio into the room so he could listen to rock and roll. Little things like that. He wanted a fan. We located a fan on another floor. These little comfort measures. I think he was very afraid of dying alone, and even though I was just his nurse, it meant something to him.

If we were to try to formalize this paradigm case in abstractions describing the nurse-patient relationship or the processes of the nurse's clinical judgments, the important meaning would be, in large measure, lost. While our efforts to formalize the process of nursing care are important to the educational endeavor, we must avoid our tendency to equate them with the concern(s) of practice that we are trying to represent.

We have much to learn from practice and from experts in practice. Now when I think of curriculum revolution, I do not think of developing more elegant and detailed formal models to be passed on to the next generation of nurses, for them to take and apply in their practice. Rather, I am struggling with ways in which the concerns of practice can truly be addressed by our educational activities, where classroom learning might be the application of practice rather than the other way around. I hope that you will join me in this struggle.

References

Benner, P. (1984). *From novice to expert: Power and excellence in nursing practice.* Menlo Park, CA: Addison-Wesley.

Benner, P. (1983). Uncovering the knowledge embedded in clinical practice. *Image: The Journal of Nursing Scholarship, 15*(2), 36-41.

Benner, P., & Tanner, C. (1987). Clinical judgment: How expert nurses use intuition. *American Journal of Nursing, 87*, 23-31.

Benner, P., & Wrubel, J. (1982). Skilled clinical knowledge: The value of perceptual awareness. *Nurse Educator, 7*(3), 11-17.

Carper, B. A. (1978). Fundamental patterns of knowing in nursing. *Advances in Nursing Science, 1*(1), 13-23.

Cianfrani, K. L. (1984). The influence of amounts and relevance of data on identifying health problems. In M. J. Kim, G. K. McFarland, & A. M. McLane (Eds.), *Classification of nursing diagnoses: Proceedings of the fifth national conference* (pp. 159-161). St. Louis, MO: Mosby.

Corcoran, S. (l986a). Task complexity and nursing expertise as factors in decision making. *Nursing Research, 35,* 107-112.

Corcoran, S. (1986b). Planning by expert and novice nurses in cases of varying complexity. *Research in Nursing and Health, 9,* 155-162.

Dreyfus, H. L. (1979). *What computers can t do: The limits of artificial intelligence.* New York: Harper & Row.

Dreyfus, H. L., & Dreyfus, S. E. (1986). *Mind over machine.* New York: Free Press.

Elstein, A., Shulman, L., & Sprafka, S. (1978). *Medical problem solving.* Cambridge, MA: MIT Press.

Gordon, M. (1980). Predictive strategies in diagnostic tasks. *Nursing Research, 29,* 39-44.

Grier, M. (1976). Decision making about patient care. *Nursing Research, 25*(2), 105-110.

Hammond, K. R., Kelly, K. J., Schneider, R. J., & Vancini, M. (1967). Clinical inference in nursing: Revising judgments. *Nursing Research, 16,* 38-45.

Heidegger, M. (1962). *Being and time* (J. Macquarrie & E. Robinson, Trans.). New York: Harper & Row. (Original work published 1927)

Matthews, C. A., & Gaul, A. L. (1979). Nursing diagnosis from the perspective of concept attainment. *Advances in Nursing Science, 2,* 17-26.

Munhall, P. L. (1982). Nursing philosophy and nursing science: In apposition or opposition. *Nursing Research, 31,* 176-177, 181.

Newell, A., & Simon, H. (1972). *Human problem solving.* Englewood Cliffs, NJ: Prentice-Hall.

Oiler, C. (1982). The phenomenological approach in nursing research. *Nursing Research, 31,*178-181.

Phillips, L. R., & Rempusheski, V. F. (1985). Diagnosing and intervening for elder abuse and neglect: An empirically generated decision-making model. *Nursing Research, 34,* 134-139.

Polanyi, M. (1958). *Personal knowledge.* Chicago: University of Chicago Press.

Pyles, S. H., & Stern, P. N. (1983). Discovery of nursing gestalt in critical care nursing: The importance of the gray gorilla syndrome. *Image: The Journal of Nursing Scholarship, 15*(2), 51-57.

Schein, E. (1973). *Professional education.* New York: McGraw-Hill.

Schon, D. A. (1983). *The reflective practitioner.* New York: Basic Books.

Tanner, C. A. (1987). Teaching clinical judgment. In J. J. Fitzpatrick & R. L. Tauton (Eds.), *Annual review of nursing research, Vol. 5* (pp. 153-173). New York: Springer Publishing.

Tanner, C. A., Padrick, K. P., Westfall, U. E., & Putzier, D. J. (1987). Diagnostic reasoning strategies of nurses and nursing students. *Nursing Research*, *36*(6), 358-363.

Westfall, U. E., Tanner, C. A., Putzier, D. J., & Padrick, K. P. (1986). Clinical inference in nursing: A preliminary analysis of cognitive strategies. *Research in Nursing and Health*, *9*, 269-277.

The Practice Mandate – 20 Years Later

Christine A. Tanner

When I wrote *The Practice Mandate* in 1988, I was deeply concerned about a number of issues emanating from our status as a practice discipline. First, it was becoming increasingly apparent that in our effort to become a research-based, scientifically oriented discipline, we often underprivileged the knowledge gained in practice – that is, the skilled know-how that escapes formalization, and because it is highly contextually bound and elicited in particular situations, could never be subject to the more highly valued empirical testing. Second, we persistently framed our curricula around abstract concepts, which failed to capture the realities of particular practice situations. I was concerned that nursing diagnoses would (however inadvertently) cloud our understanding of the patient's situation, concerns, and health issues rather than clearly communicate them, and that nursing process as a framework for clinical judgment failed to capture, and in some ways obscured, what students need to learn to be able to think like a nurse. At that time, we had yet to develop curricula that captured ways in which faculty could bring the realities of clinical practice – practical knowledge, a deep understanding of patients' concerns, and skillful clinical judgment – into the classroom.

In the intervening years, there has been significant scholarly work about the nature of nursing knowledge and clinical judgment in nursing practice. In an integrative review of the literature of more than 190 studies on clinical judgment (Tanner, 2006), I drew the following conclusions:

> *Evidence suggests that skilled clinical judgment is case based, contextually bound, interpretive reasoning rather than the instrumental application of scientifically based knowledge to the resolution of problems, as suggested by the nursing process.*

> *Clinical judgments are more influenced by what the nurse brings to the situation than the objective data about the situation at hand. Deep background knowledge is essential for setting up expectations of what will be seen in each clinical case, for noticing the unexpected, for considering plausible interpretations, for collecting reasonable evidence, for choosing the best course of action.*

> *Every clinical judgment has an ethical component, in that judgment is shaped by a deep understanding of the patient s experience, and a vision for what makes excellent care.*

Since the time of the Curriculum Revolution, nurse educators have zealously adopted critical thinking as an outcome of nursing education programs, but virtually every published work on critical thinking points to the confusion of terminology and the conflation of clinical judgment with critical thinking. Research indicates that critical thinking and clinical judgment are **not** the same constructs. I believe nurse educators want their graduates to have general critical thinking skills, that is, to be able recognize and analyze assumptions, challenge the status quo, evaluate limitations in health care, and take action to improve it. This kind of critical thinking embodies a different set of dispositions and thinking skills than what we mean when we think about clinical judgment in patient care.

A better understanding of both critical thinking and clinical judgment would greatly influence our educational practices. It would encourage interest in narrative pedagogy and in case-based instructional approaches. And it would demand new approaches to clinical education. For example, when faculty rely on the nursing process and the ever-present nursing care plan, they decontextualize nursing judgments and emphasize scientific rationale. To better teach clinical judgment, faculty must emphasize the narrative nature of reasoning, coaching students in the consideration of the general rule in relation to the particular case.

In the intervening years, the science of learning has advanced tremendously; we know a great deal more about how people learn, and what instructional approaches are likely to enhance learning. For example, Chickering and Gamson (1991) used several decades of educational research to derive seven principles of good practice in undergraduate education. They indicate that good teaching practice:

1. encourages contacts between students and faculty,

2. develops reciprocity and cooperation among students,

3. encourages active learning,

4. gives prompt feedback,

5. emphasizes time on task,

6. communicates high expectations, and

7. respects diverse talents and ways of learning.

Several other recent key works summarize the tremendous literature on learning, extrapolating significant lessons for college faculty (e.g., Bransford, Brown, & Cocking, 2004; Weimer, 2002). These are core ideas promoted during the Curriculum Revolution that have gained legitimacy as higher education has sought to renew emphasis on its teaching mission and on the paradigm shift from teaching to learning.

In these same intervening years, nursing and related science have grown exponentially, and the content that students are expected to master has become overwhelming for both students and teachers. Nurse educators feel enormous pressures from both students and colleagues to *cover* content (NLN, 2003). Yet we know that the deep learning needed for skilled clinical practice requires much more than superficial content coverage. Deep learning requires time to think, reflect on, connect with previous learning and extend in clinical practice.

As Ironside (2003a) has astutely pointed out, the challenge for nurse educators is to find ways to overcome the focus on covering content at the expense of engaging students in thinking.

And in these same intervening years, nursing practice has changed profoundly both in predicted and unexpected ways, fueled largely by shifting economics of health care, changing demographics, and a rapidly encroaching shortage of nurses. We have witnessed a tremendous increase in the complexity and acuity of patient care in the hospital setting, decreased lengths of stay, the shift of care and recovery to the home and community, and an explosion of new technologies. Yet despite these changes, clinical education has changed very little. Nurse educators continue to struggle with our time-honored approaches to clinical education (one faculty member supervising 8-10 students). Except in our most innovative nursing programs, we continue to use, in Porter-O'Grady's terms, "resident, bed-based nursing care fundamentals as the foundation for basic nursing education" (2001, p. 183). From fundamentals on, students are placed in a clinical setting, where they can be assigned to a patient, develop a plan of care applying what they have learned in their theory courses, and provide total patient care based on that care plan. The learning is derived from students acting like nurses, learning from providing care to one or more patients each week and absorbing whatever other learning presents itself while in the clinical setting (Tanner, 2002). Of course, there are minor variations in the structure of this experience, but the core of the clinical experience is the "case assignment." As reported in a recent survey, 98% of baccalaureate nursing programs require students to write care plans as a significant part of their clinical experiences (Chappy & Stewart, 2004). Coupled with a senior preceptorship, concentrated at the end of the program, the case assignment method occupies the majority of the clinical experiences within any given program.

The Curriculum Revolution of the 1980s was, in large measure, a critique of the behavioral pedagogy that dominated nursing education, limiting the vision of nurse educators and keeping us trapped in the content-driven, mechanistic approaches to education. Our hope was that through our uncovering and critique of the taken-for-granted assumptions of behavioral pedagogy, we could empower nurse educators to develop pedagogies more appropriate for a practice discipline that is populated by caring, critically thinking practitioners. At the time, we did not offer an alternative pedagogy. Since then, new pedagogies have emerged. For example, the work of Nancy Diekelmann and her colleagues (Diekelmann, 2001; Ironside, 2005, 2006; Scheckel & Ironside, 2006) in narrative pedagogy has been implemented in several schools and has been successful in carrying forward the ideals of the Curriculum Revolution (Andrews, et al., 2001; Diekelmann, 2001; Ironside, 2003a, 2003b, 2006).

Were I to write a "practice mandate" paper today, I would continue to raise the concerns of two decades ago, challenging faculty to deepen our understanding of what it is to think like a nurse and to find ways to bring clinical practice to the classroom. But I would add two significant items to the practice mandate agenda:

- Fundamental reform in our clinical education in ways that a) purposefully support the development and integration of clinical thinking, action, and skillful ethical comportment, b) incorporate an understanding of how students develop over time in their clinical acumen, and c) make better use of our limited clinical sites.

- Fundamental reform of the nursing curriculum to more closely align with the changing health care needs of the people we serve and to address the issues raised in recent accounts of the health care quality chasm and patient safety (IOM, 2001). Nursing should be at the forefront of health promotion and chronic illness management, yet I think we would be hard-pressed to show where in our prelicensure programs nursing students are getting the education that prepares them for such practice. The IOM reports and subsequent work on patient safety clearly outline new, significant competencies that should be expected of all health professional students – extending the practice mandate for a curriculum revolution (IOM, 2001, 2004; AACN, 2006).

It would be tempting to declare that transformation of nursing education in the current context of faculty shortages and other scarce resources as "Mission Impossible". But I believe that the opposite is true. It is my sense that the rapid changes in health care, the shifting population needs, and the acute nursing shortage have catalyzed fundamental change, perhaps the most profound in our recent history. The first steps of that transformation are becoming increasingly apparent as nursing faculty begin to challenge their long-standing, taken-for-granted assumptions; as they set aside differences and their internecine warfare of the entry-into-practice debates; as they begin stronger and deeper collaborations with their clinical partners.

We won't see the evidence of these changes in the literature for a while, because they are just getting started and data are still being collected. Nonetheless, there are some promising initiatives of the major transformation we seek. For example, the Oregon Consortium for Nursing Education (OCNE) has resulted from unprecedented collaboration between community college and university faculty, with an eye to develop a standard, competency-based curriculum to prepare the "new" nurse, and to improve access to a seamless baccalaureate curriculum (Gubrud-Howe, et al., 2003; OCNE, 2007). The first students were enrolled in nursing courses fall semester of 2006 on eight campuses – the four campuses of Oregon Health Sciences University and four community colleges, with two additional community college campuses admitting students in 2007 and two more in 2008. In this curriculum, fundamentals of nursing have been redefined as evidence-based practice, culturally sensitive and relationship-centered care, leadership, and clinical judgment, with these concepts and others introduced early and spiraled throughout the curriculum. Through a two-year faculty development program, faculty leaders in the OCNE partner programs have taken to heart the many lessons about learning, intentionally attending to content selection that will help reduce the volume while focusing on the most prevalent health conditions. Instructional approaches have been tremendously changed, with an emphasis on case-based instruction, integrating distance delivery technologies, and using simulation, drawing on best practices in the development of these approaches (Billings, Connors, & Skiba, 2001; Issenberg, et al., 2005; Jeffries, 2005). OCNE leaders obtained funding from Kaiser Permanente Northwest to begin the long, collaborative, consensus-building process to transform clinical education. Evaluation has and will continue to be an integral part of this work, with an eye to adding to our collective knowledge of best practices in nursing education.

We see evidence of similar efforts, mostly state or regional, in order to build on prior alliances, acknowledge geographic particularities, and respond to local needs in many other parts of the country, from Hawaii to New Jersey, Texas to Montana. The nursing shortage has been a primary catalyst. It has captured the interest of potential funders, from individual donors and foundations to the federal government. The keys are collaboration and a collective voice for nursing, a willingness to work through long-standing and divisive issues, and, most importantly, a moral commitment to the populations we serve.

References

American Association of Colleges of Nursing. (2006). *Hallmarks of quality and patient safety: Recommended baccalaureate competencies and curricular guidelines to assure high quality and safe patient care*. Retrieved November 15, 2006 from http://www.aacn.nche.edu/Education/pdf/PSHallmarks9-06.pdf

Andrews, C. A., Ironside, P. M., Nosek, C., Sims, S. L., Swenson, M. M., Yeomans, C., et al. (2001). Enacting narrative pedagogy: The lived experiences of students and teachers. *Nursing and Health Care Perspectives, 22*(5), 252-259.

Billings, D. M., Connors, H. R., & Skiba, D. J. (2001). Benchmarking best practices in web-based nursing courses. *Advances in Nursing Science, 23*(3), 41-52.

Bransford, J. D., Brown, A. L. & Cocking, R. R. (Eds.). (2004). *How people learn*. Washington, DC: National Academy Press.

Chappy, S. L. & Stewart, S. (2004). Curricular practices in baccalaureate nursing education: Results of a national survey. *Journal of Professional Nursing, 20*, 369-373.

Chickering, A. W. & Gamson, Z. F. (1991). Applying the seven principles of good practice in undergraduate education. In *New Directions for Teaching & Learning*, (No. 47). San Francisco: Jossey-Bass.

Diekelmann, N. L. (2001). Narrative pedagogy: Heideggerian hermeneutical analyses of lived experiences of students, teachers, and clinicians. *Advances in Nursing Science, 23*(3), 53-71.

Gubrud-Howe, P., Shaver, K. S., Tanner, C. A., Bennett-Stillmaker, J., Davidson, S. B., Flaherty-Robb, M., et al. (2003). A challenge to meet the future: Nursing education in Oregon, 2010. *Journal of Nursing Education, 42*(4), 163-167.

Institute of Medicine. (2001). *Crossing the quality chasm*. Washington, DC: National Academies Press.

Institute of Medicine. (2004). *Keeping patients safe: Transforming the work environment of nurses*. Washington, DC: National Academies Press.

Ironside, P. M. (2003a). New pedagogies for teaching thinking: The lived experiences of students and teachers enacting Narrative Pedagogy. *Journal of Nursing Education, 42,* 509-516.

Ironside, P. M. (2003b). Trying something new: Implementing and evaluating narrative pedagogy using a multimethod approach. *Nursing Education Perspectives, 24,* 122-128.

Ironside, P. M. (2005). Teaching thinking and reaching the limits of memorization: Enacting new pedagogies. *Journal of Nursing Education, 44,* 441-449.

Ironside, P. M. (2006). Using narrative pedagogy: Learning and practicing interpretive thinking. *Journal of Advanced Nursing, 55,* 478-486.

Issenberg, S. B., McGaghie, W. C., Petrusa, E. R., Gordon, D. L., & Scalese, R. J. (2005). Features and uses of high fidelity medical simulations that lead to effective learning: A BEME systematic review. *Medical Teacher, 27*(1), 10-28.

Jeffries, P. R. (2005). A framework for designing, implementing, and evaluating simulations used as teaching strategies in nursing. *Nursing Education Perspectives, 26*(2), 96-103.

National League for Nursing. (2003). *Position statement. Innovation in nursing education: A call to reform.* Retrieved November 13, 2006, from http://www.nln.org/aboutnln/PositionStatements/innovation.htm

OCNE, 2006. Update on Progress. Retrieved July 11, 2007 from http://www.ocne.org/update.php

Porter-O'Grady, T. (2001). Profound change: 21st century nursing. *Nursing Outlook, 49,* 182-186.

Scheckel, M. M., & Ironside, P. M. (2006). Enacting Narrative Pedagogy: Cultivating interpretive thinking. *Nursing Outlook, 54,* 159-165.

Tanner, C. A. (2002). Clinical education, circa 2010. *Journal of Nursing Education, 41,* 51-52.

Tanner, C. A. (2006). Thinking like a nurse: A research based model of clinical judgment in nursing. *Journal of Nursing Education, 45,* 204-211.

Weimer, M. E. (2002). *Learner centered teaching: Five key changes to practice*. San Francisco: Jossey-Bass.

Critical Social Theory and Nursing Education[1]

David G. Allen

Introduction

My goal in this chapter is to suggest some implications of critical social theory for nursing education. To do this, I will first develop a brief analogy between critical theory and the idea of informed consent. Following this analogy will be a short explication of critical theory as a philosophical position. I will then address the application of critical theory to nursing education by exploring how it changes the way educators view students. The implications of this altered view of the student-as-person for both curricular and pedagogical approaches will be suggested through examples of classroom practices and faculty decision making.

This movement between the abstract and the more concrete is a strategy I will use throughout this chapter, partly because of the lack of exposure to critical theory in nursing, but primarily because I want to stress that critical theory is an eminently practical enterprise.

What Critical Theory Is

At heart, critical theory is a theory of social rationality, of how communities or groups make "rational" decisions. It is not a method, although it has implications for method. It also is not a recommendation for any particular social arrangement – liberal democracy or socialism, for example – although it has implications for social formations.

Let me preface my philosophical explication with an analogy between informed consent (a more familiar model of social rationality) and critical theory (Allen, 1987a). As the technical and invasive basis of medicine exploded, it became clear that patients were undergoing hazardous treatments with relatively uncertain outcomes. When these patients suffered the consequences of these treatments – including both failure to cure and morbidity of side effects – they raised the question of whether, had they truly realized the possible consequences, they would have chosen to undergo the treatment.

Our procedures for informed consent, whatever their limitations, were developed because we health professionals and advocates believed that not all consent was "informed," or rational. In an effort to counterbalance the authority of physicians and the tremendous difference in medical knowledge between physicians and patients, formal informed consent procedures were developed.

---

1. Originally presented at the first National Conference on Nursing Education in Chicago and published in *Curriculum revolution: Redefining the student-teacher relationship* (1990, pp. 67-86). New York: National League for Nursing. Reprinted with permission.

I am not suggesting these procedures work. What I want to emphasize is that we developed a formal process or set of procedures to try to insure that these important decisions were made on as rational a basis as possible. We did not try to replace the current model of medicine with, for example, socialized medicine or a return to midwives or lay healers – although there are rational advocates for these positions. Our intent was to shape the process by which medical decisions were made so that we could be reasonably comfortable that people understood their options.

The intent behind informed consent is similar to the intent behind critical theory. A community makes many important decisions, including what form of government it will adopt, what will count as authoritative scientific or religious knowledge, and whether and how it will use risky technology such as nuclear energy. What critical theory attempts to articulate is what *principles* should be in operation if these important decisions are to be rational.

In nursing education we face similar decisions. How should we organize our schools? What knowledge will we present as legitimate? How will we know if students are making rational choices concerning their education and nursing care? How do we encourage, persuade, or compel students to adopt our views of nursing and how will we know when they have embraced them as their own? Critical theory offers a perspective on how to approach these vital concerns.

Critical Theory as a Philosophical Perspective

Throughout history, communities have wrestled with questions such as the ones I briefly outlined. In seeking a basis for deciding between options, they have appealed to different standards of rationality. For example, in some communities the option that best corresponded to the teachings of a spiritual leader or a sacred text was the option chosen. Empiricism shifted authority away from the church or state toward a more democratic foundation – the contents of experience that were presumably available to everyone, not just priests or kings (Harding, 1986).

As Thomas Kuhn (1962) attempted to articulate, the authority of empiricism has neither extraterrestrial nor ahistoric, transcendental foundations. The standards of scientific rationality, however, are grounded in the historically contingent values and decisions of scientific communities. Changes in scientific values – such as the ones currently being discussed concerning nursing research – are not best viewed as advances in rationality or the progressive deciphering of nature's own language. Rather, they are reasonable choices of which scientific vocabularies seem most effective for a given set of purposes. After all, no observation could possibly justify using observation as a truth criterion (Bernstein, 1983). At least for a while though, observation was seen as a more effective criterion for choosing between alternative theories than divine revelation or the opinion of a cabinet minister.

It may be fair to characterize contemporary philosophy of science as primarily a debate about 1) whether any ahistoric, transcendental foundation or criterion is possible, 2) if it is not, then what are the alternatives besides self-contradictory relativism or historicism, and 3) if such a foundation is possible, what is it and why have all previous attempts to establish one turned out to be futile and often politically and scientifically regressive? Another way of putting this is that it is a debate between *foundationists,* those who believe there is some such criterion, and that this criterion is grounded in a reality that is not dependent on social conventions, and *antifoundationists,* those who believe such a criterion is a chimera that serves chiefly to institutionalize one group's view as Truth with a capital T (Benhabib, 1986; White, 1988).

Critical theory, as I am employing it, falls within the *anti*foundationist camp. Perhaps it is best seen as agnostic on the question of foundations. What it asserts is that even if we decide there is such a foundation, what is essential is to insure that such a decision is as rational as possible. Thus, critical theory is basically a theory of communicative rationality (Habermas, 1984, 1987). It is a theory about what principles underlie our collective decision making.

Since I believe that in our culture education is important, if for no other reason than that the students we educate will have to make a decision about foundationism, then it seems to me that critical theory has some exciting possibilities for nursing education. Thus, I will now briefly describe some of the central tenets of critical theory and their implications for nursing education.

Critical Theory and Nursing Education

Let me begin by outlining some issues in nursing education to which critical theory might speak.

Accreditation

What criteria should we use to identify competent nursing education? More importantly, how should we decide which criteria to use? If the criteria about what constitutes science and authoritative knowledge are being hotly contested, how can we decide the criteria for education? Note I assume we cannot and should not evade the obligation to make such decisions. If, as many philosophers of science and ethics increasingly argue, such decisions are grounded in community, what is the community of nursing? Should regional or religious nursing communities develop their own criteria? *Are students part of the nursing community?*

Curriculum

Even setting aside the question of accreditation, many of us struggle with how to make reasonable decisions about how to organize learning (Pitts, 1985). Increasingly dissatisfied with education guided by what my colleagues refer to as "dropping students into the middle of a lake and telling them to swim to all shores at the same time" or "assembling them in auditoriums and hosing them down with microfacts," we are questioning the very criteria we use. It no longer seems feasible to define a "generalist" as someone having exposure to, or even some knowledge of, the dizzying array of specialties or content areas in nursing (Diekelmann, 1990).

Again, the implications of critical theory for this debate are not so much related to which particular options we choose but under what communicative conditions we make that choice. It feels increasingly unreasonable to spend precious time rearranging the deck chairs of course content on the Titanic of nursing education (Diekelmann, Allen, & Tanner, 1989).

Teaching

One of the delights of contemporary nursing students is their diversity: they come to us as men, women, workers, parents, minorities, gays, lesbians – all with different histories and aspirations. Is our goal to somehow acknowledge such incoming diversity while trying to meld it into a single image of the graduating nurse (Giroux, 1988)? Is such diversity merely incidental to being a nurse? How, in a single classroom, do I facilitate the unpartnered 19-year-old white woman who decided to be a nurse when she was eight years old and the 40-year-old woman of color who wants to support her two school-age children?

Having so briefly sketched what I believe to be some fundamental issues in nursing education, let me tie them to the preceding introduction to critical theory by linking some central precepts of critical theory to a view of the nursing student-as-person.

Central Concepts of Critical Theory

In this section I will discuss three sets of concepts: 1) autonomy and responsibility; 2) essentialism and subjectivity, and 3) the technical, practical, and emancipatory interests of nursing education.

Autonomy and Responsibility

Given the need to make important decisions in a nursing community, in a context of communicative action, critical theory identifies two principles that must guide interaction in order to maximize rationality. These are "autonomy" and "responsibility," and I wish I could say them as one word because they are inseparable. Many people believe a central malady in American culture is their separation and the privileging of autonomy over responsibility. Let me explain. The context I am working in, remember, is the necessity to insure that important community decisions, such as those about science, nursing education, or nuclear power, are as rational as possible when there is no "higher authority" to appeal to.

Autonomy refers to the principle that should guide me as an individual to speak without internal or external constraints. If the group is to make a good decision, the members should be able to count on me sharing my views and not restricting my participation either because of internal constraints, such as fear of public speaking or self-doubts as to my intelligence, or because of external constraints such as threat of censure or loss of employment. If I don't speak because of these constraints, I may withhold a vital piece to the puzzle that the group will never hear. Consequently, the ultimate decision may be less than optimal (Habermas, 1984).

The principle of responsibility refers to my commitment to the speaking community to insure that others can speak with the same autonomy I do. If I intimidate through masculine speaking strategies or see someone else being inhibited from speaking, I have a responsibility to nurture that person's willingness to participate and prevent others from blocking participation. Responsibility furthers self-interest, because I have a vital interest in the group making the best decision. It may be that a poor black woman, against whom countless constraints operate, has the clearest idea about how we should proceed (even if she discounts her own view) (Nicolson, 1989).

As a teacher I struggle with this issue in seminars and small group discussions. I require participation and include peer and instructor evaluation of participation in all small classes. My rationale, which I explain to students, is that "being quiet" is not just an issue of personal style, it is parasitic of the group. When a member of the class has the benefit of everyone else's perspectives on the issue, but the group doesn't get to hear that individual's insights, the group members are deprived of information that may help them come to a more complete understanding. Commitment to group understanding is a central educational value. I also recognize that everyone has a responsibility to nurture and support people to facilitate their participation.

The reason I say I struggle with this requirement is that the classroom speaking situation is structured by teacher-student power imbalances. In my case, this is often complicated by my being a male teacher in a class comprised primarily, or entirely, of women (Pagano, 1988; Culley & Portuges, 1985). The best compromise I have been able to work out is to make my rationale explicit and leave this "requirement" – as with all requirements – open for negotiation.

This play of gender and power in teaching brings me to the next set of concepts: essentialism and subjectivity.

Essentialism and Subjectivity

Under this heading, the main point concerns our conceptualization of students as people. The term "subjectivity" refers to the interplay of social history and individual initiative in creating human experience. "Essentialism" may be an unfamiliar term, but it is related to the notion of foundationism that I discussed earlier (Allen, 1986a). The antifoundationist, remember, argues that there is no simple, ahistoric, nonsocial, transcendental criterion as to what constitutes science or rational or authoritative knowledge. Rather, these criteria shift historically and only emerge at times of "normal science" as a consensus within a scientific community. In other words, scientific criteria are contextually defined; they are shaped by the context, including the intended purposes, in which they emerge. Another way to put this is to say there is no "essence" of science. What counts as science changes over time.

When the same critique of "essences" (i.e., that they don't exist) is applied to the notion of persons or "subjects," we arrive at a view supported by symbolic interactionists that there is no "essential self or singular identity;" in different situations we are different people. Without going into the complex rethinking of language and subjectivity that led to this position, let me try to indicate what I mean using myself as an example.

Under the central social categories of gender, race, class, and sexual orientation, I am a white, upper-middle-class, professional, heterosexual male. These categories, these aspects of myself, my "subjectivity," converge and conflict in interesting ways. Since social opportunities and resources are distributed according to these categories, my whiteness brings me certain advantages over people of color, my maleness privileges me over women, my professionalism is a form of occupational dominance, and my heterosexualism protects my intimacy needs and my access to tax breaks and employment benefits (Allen, 1986b; Allen & Wolfgram, 1988).

In many situations, however, these categories conflict; men benefit from the economic segregation of women in low paying fields such as nursing, and yet I am a nurse. My white maleness may align me with black males or white females depending on whether the issue is perpetuation of pornography – which favors men, including black men – or access to higher education, which privileges whites, including white women. Further, all these categories change over time. (Masculinity in the 1980s is not the same as masculinity was in the 1890s, no matter how much my feminist friends despair over the similarities.)

The point here is not so much autobiographical as theoretical. I participate in meaning systems around gender, race, and class. I understand myself, my self-interests, my goals differently in different situations. In contemporary jargon, this is referred to as being a "split subject." We are all "split" into these different categories; there is no unifying essence or core criterion by which I can establish who I am (Allen, Allman, & Powers, 1990). This split becomes problematic when a single situation calls forth conflicting aspects. Being an adult male in nursing school or a single mother working in construction are examples in which there is no unified response. To be a nursing student, I must at times deny my adultness and masculinity; to be a construction worker may make problematic one's femininity and motherhood.

A more familiar model of split subjects is found in Freudian theory. Freud has experienced somewhat of a rebirth in social theory, although not because of his specific conclusions about oedipal conflicts or penis envy. Instead of these problematic conclusions, what people find helpful in Freud is a model of how social conflicts become part of our identity, our consciousness. Our needs, both conscious and unconscious, are as socially constructed as our beliefs about religion and science (Allen, 1985). Different and conflicting desires are created from birth – for example, the desire for intimacy and oneness and the desire for autonomy. We are often unaware of these conflicting desires until we are in a situation that calls up both but can satisfy only one.

Common examples are found in the work of many feminist theorists when they discuss tensions in intimate relationships between men and women (e.g., Rose, 1983). A more concrete example is the value our culture puts on self-expression and individualism at the same time that workplaces are increasingly routinized and bureaucratized. Instead of seeking self-realization in work, people are now encouraged to find it in consumption – which is itself the acquisition of mass-produced items, the ownership of which is supposed to secure individual identity. In nursing, we find that people enter the field visualizing nursing as a one-to-one helping relationship, while profit-oriented delivery organizations, the nursing shortage, and increasing acuity seem to call for less individualized care (Reverby, 1987).

Such conflicts are neither escapable nor undesirable from a critical theory of education perspective. Situations in which these conflicting desires are called forth – both in the classroom and in clinical sites – can be opportunities for students and faculty to become conscious of these conflicts and study them (Misgeld, 1985; Freire, 1986, 1987). For example, the discomfort of an elderly female patient with me, as a male, supervising a student's efforts at catheterizing her can be the occasion to discuss how nursing as a gendered social relationship exists in tension with a view of nursing as a gender-neutral science. This tension was discussed a few years ago in regard to a lawsuit brought by a male nurse who was not permitted to work in ob/gyn because the hospital could not guarantee that a patient who did not want to be attended by a man would not have this man assigned to her. I argued that the asymmetry of gender relationships outside the hospital, where women are subject to the constant threat of sexual abuse, could not be simply "left outside," but that they shaped interactions between nurse and patient regardless of the technical skill of the male nurse involved.

Similarly, peer-led discussions in small classes about why the students became interested in nursing often reveal that many students are the children of alcoholics and/or have been sexually abused. Discussions of the similarities between the literature on adult children of alcoholics, the literature on women's invisible work, and many students' ideas of nursing can produce profitable insights into the constraints and possibilities these childhood experiences create. A colleague of mine believes some of the incapacitating anxiety we see in some nursing students is symptomatic of conflicts around bodies and vulnerability.

So far in this section, I have explained how communicative rationality depends on the twin principles of autonomy and responsibility. From these principles and the complexity of their instantiation in teaching, I moved to an explanation of subjectivity via the notion of split subjects. In turn, I hope this view of subjectivity helped highlight how discourses of gender, race, and class mold communicative activity.

In the next section on the social interests guiding education, I hope to link these themes in an analysis of several practices in nursing education.

Technical, Practical, and Emancipatory Interests

In the context of discussing the fact that science is not value neutral and that different approaches to science are guided by different values, Jurgen Habermas, the leading critical theorist, identified three *interests* that underlie science (Habermas, 1979; Allen, 1985). These interests are 1) technical, 2) practical, and 3) emancipatory. My theme in this section is that these three interests can also be seen to underlie education and that problems emerge, as they do in science, when we fail to identify and debate which interest is operating. Each entails a very different image of the student-as-person.

Technical Interests. The social interest underlying technical science and technically oriented education is prediction and control. Technical interest is shaped by a means-end relationship. Once the ends are established, or, more often, assumed or asserted by "experts," the quest becomes seeking the best way to accomplish them, i.e., to control the situation in order to produce the predicted outcome.

This view undergirds what Em Bevis refers to as the "training model" of nursing education. We, the experts, decide what "product" we want, specify the competencies we want to instill, the kind of nurse we want to graduate, and then conduct research or develop programs to produce the desired results. The criteria for selecting among competing means are most often efficiency and effectiveness (Diekelmann, Allen, & Tanner, 1989). (I am not assuming, by the way, that we have much of a rational basis for believing the means we pick actually do produce what we intend.)

An important dimension of this process is that "experts," in this case nurse educators, identify the desired outcomes. The logic here is quite analogous to the critique I offered of the Social Policy Statement (SPS) in which the nurse "diagnoses and treats" (Allen, 1987b). We educators diagnose the problem, identify the goal, and "treat" the student in order to overcome the problem – such as a knowledge deficit or unprofessional values – in order to achieve our goal. Just as the SPS pays scant lip service to the clients' ability to determine the goal and identify acceptable means, we display minimal regard for the goals our students are pursuing and their evaluation of the means we have selected to accomplish our goal. This can be seen in practices such as fully specifying in advance the desired outcomes of a course, often as behavioral objectives. The notion of education as behavior change, which has been so thoroughly critiqued by Bevis and others, is fundamentally a technical view (Weiler, 1988).

Under the technically oriented model of education, the student is largely seen as "raw material." Diversity, while occasionally acknowledged, is viewed as a variance in the raw material to be shaped by curricular and pedagogical processes the faculty have designed with the goal of graduating a person with the attributes the faculty value. "Compliance" and "coping" are common vocabularies characterizing students. Any tension between what students "need" (as determined by faculty) and what they "want" is either ignored or viewed as a mistaken perception of self-interest (Roberts, 1983).

The histories and aspirations of the student are ignored by technical interests. It is not so much that these histories and aspirations are seen as negative, they are just considered irrelevant to the operations of education. Acknowledgment of individualism is limited, for the most part, to selections of preestablished and usually limited "electives," which must fit into a highly structured and regimented program of study.

From the perspective of critical theory, students have been banished from the speaking community. While the faculty community may work to establish conditions of autonomy and responsibility among themselves, students are not included. From an ethical perspective, they are nonpersons.

It is not, Bevis and I would argue, that technical interest has no useful place in nursing education. It is that, in the first place, its role needs to be debated and, second, it has a very limited role. I would see its role being limited to the following conditions:

1. When students agree, under conditions of autonomy and responsibility, to *both* the goal and to the acceptability of the means.

2. When students and faculty agree there is a good bit of evidence to support that the proposed means will in fact accomplish the agreed-upon goal.

For the most part, the technical model of education is best used to teach psychomotor skills. One example concerns when and how we teach technical skills. In many schools, faculty have labored, and labored in futility, to convince students that they didn't need to learn technical skills, that these were no big deal. Often the result is that, when faced with a patient whose care requires such a skill, students can attend to little else and are unable to bring to bear many of the things they have learned about nursing care.

Yet when I teach incoming students and elicit their views of nursing and what they want to learn, psychomotor skills often rank very high. Never mind that this is a "technical" rather than the favored "professional" view of nursing we educators prefer; it remains the "St. Elsewhere" [a popular T.V. drama at the time] lay definition that many students bring into school with them. Still, we pass over this opportunity to meet them "where they're at" and try instead to persuade them they shouldn't be there.

The notion of explicating students' understanding of nursing and their educational goals brings with it the next educational interest.

Practical Interests. While the concept of "technical" is familiar to us, it is a mark of our culture that we have lost the distinction between the technical and the practical. The practical is the realm of everyday communicative interaction in which *understanding* is the central interest. Understanding is necessary if we are to orient ourselves to the pursuit of shared goals (Diekelmann, 1990). Communicative action of a practical nature presupposes, in the act of conversation, the values of autonomy and responsibility. If conversation is genuinely oriented toward understanding, it must have as its presupposition that I am speaking my mind as openly as I can and am expecting and facilitating the same from my conversational partner.

Arriving at this understanding is sometimes called a "fusion of horizons." This simply means that we all enter a conversation with a taken-for-granted background or "horizon" that shapes and makes possible the interpretation of what each of us means. The important contribution Martin Heidegger, and especially Hans Georg Gadamer, made to our grasp of communication is that we can never stand outside this "horizon" and, even if it were possible, doing so would block any comprehension at all. What is required is bringing the shared and separate aspects of our horizons together (Thompson, 1990).

Critical theory identifies two dimensions that underlie such an agreed understanding. There is "normatively secured" consensus, in which agreement is made possible by jointly held values and beliefs. Thus in a religious community, educational decisions are grounded in this shared normative basis. "Communicatively achieved" consensus occurs when the normative validity claims on which agreement depends are themselves "on the table" to be discussed, clarified, and agreed upon. If we share a context in which these assumptions do not inhibit understanding, we may progress in our conversation. This chapter is directed at trying to put some of these normative dimensions of our educational decisions "on the table" for debate in order to create a communicatively achieved consensus about values associated with the student-as-person.

The central task in the practical domain, then, is a hermeneutic or interpretive one. The goal is to clarify the meaning of your conversational partner's message as well as your own. It's important to stress here that in this context hermeneutics is nonfoundational. There is no "real" or "single, fixed" meaning. Agreement on meaning is an achievement that is accomplished in a specific context and may need renegotiation as the context changes.

I believe that interpretive skills are fundamental to the development of a coherent nursing education. We pay varying degrees of attention to this when we encourage students to develop an understanding of a client's perspective on their illness and its treatment. In my experience, however, most schools spend relatively little time developing such skills.

For example, almost all BSN programs have a required research course. Part of the rationale for such a course is the need to place and reinforce nursing as having a scientific foundation. An accompanying assumption is that one avenue toward securing more professional autonomy is the scientific demonstration of nursing's efficacy. I would suggest that the individual and collective powerlessness our clinicians continue to experience is based far less on the absence of research than on the absence of hermeneutic and rhetorical skills. We might try replacing research courses with courses in how to analyze verbal interactions and formulate and deliver effective, persuasive rationales. Facility with a scientific vocabulary is an important dimension of persuasive strategies in health care settings, but in the first place it has a relatively minor role and in the second, I don't find we teach students how to use a scientific vocabulary in actual speaking situations.

In a similar vein, several colleagues with whom I have taught graduate courses on philosophy of science and feminist theory have discovered that students are fairly powerless (and often angry) when faced with theoretical discourses. While they have learned how to read scientific reports, often they can say little more than they agree or disagree with a theoretical argument. They are relatively unable to explicate, critique, and defend a theoretical position. We now begin these courses with a section on how to read and analyze arguments. Such skills are basic to the type of discourse that shapes public and organizational decisions (Allen, Bowers, & Diekelmann, 1989).

The ability to analyze discourse and to clarify or critique the assumptions embedded in one's cultural tradition are basic to a wide range of activities. The absence of this ability leads to the technical pseudo-talk that so characterized our last presidential election. These lessons can be built into nursing education in several ways. One avenue is through the humanities, the disciplines that focus directly on explicating and transmitting tradition. Most of our BSN students graduate with a series of introductory humanities courses, leaving them with freshman-level skills. A serious reexamination of our failure to *educate* rather than train students must include, as Jean Watson has said, a rebalancing of humanities with natural and social sciences.

The upsurge of the writing-to-learn and critical thinking movements suggests these abilities can be nurtured in nursing courses as well. Reconceptualizing writing assignments away from the mechanical recording of predigested information and toward discovery and articulation of insight is one avenue to explore. [The Curriculum Revolution] will suggest many possible alternatives.

The practical model of education requires a shift away from the technical view of the student as raw material forged into shape under the hammer and anvil of the value-neutral nurse educator. Our students come to us as full persons with histories that are no less complex than our own. Social contradictions in our cultural meaning systems will cause them to be borne along as split subjects with contradictory goals just as we educators are.

Achievement of understanding between faculty and students must be a mutual process guided by the principles of autonomy and responsibility. This does not mean, as some fear, abandoning our understanding of our own beliefs and commitments. It means recognizing that these are, precisely, beliefs and commitments, not transcendental principles. Consequently, course objectives and curricular goals must be continually resecured through communicative action.

For example, students have yet to persuade me that their desire for graded clinicals outweighs the damaging tensions between inquiry and evaluation in the context of patient care. Concern for grades inevitably leads to hiding ignorance and insecurity, which is extremely problematic when the care and well being of people is at stake. My belief in ungraded clinicals is a conclusion based on the evidence, experiences, and alternatives I have explored. I remain committed to renegotiating it as these contexts change.

The notion of negotiation in the complex crucible of educational conversations shaped by power and gender differences – just as they are in health care institutions – brings us to the third educational interest.

Emancipatory Interests. Briefly revisiting the analogy of informed consent may help me set the stage for explaining emancipatory educational interests. Imagine we witness an interaction between an elderly female Medicaid patient and a young surgeon concerning his belief that the woman should have a carotid endarterectomy. He explains carefully and patiently what her problem is, what the procedure is and why he thinks it will help her. At the end of the interaction, he asks her if she has any questions, she says no and signs the consent form.

When a nurse discusses this interaction with her, she expresses some fear of the procedure and some doubts that she will survive it. When offered the option of a second opinion from a surgeon on the staff who is a woman, the patient declines. She says it is important that her doctor believes she trusts him to know what is good for her, and she would not see a female physician because "they aren't as good."

In a situation such as this, there are a number of factors operating that may lead us to question whether the consent was "rational" even though both parties did their best and may not be aware of how these factors distorted the communicative situation. The physician loves working with older patients because his grandparents provided him nurturance his physician father didn't, and because older patients are so agreeable and easy to work with. The Medicaid patient is dependent on the health care system, believes women aren't as good at making "important, scientific decisions" as men are, and doesn't think a patient should "bother" a busy physician with her "petty" questions and worries.

In this situation, both speakers are operating from assumptions and identities that block autonomy and responsibility. By failing to realize, for example, the power he asserts as a male and as a physician, the doctor fails to be responsible for creating a speaking situation that would facilitate the woman's autonomous participation. Similarly, her beliefs about her identity as a woman and her role as a patient prevent her from speaking autonomously.

Similar dynamics operate in teaching situations. Research by Barbara Bowers revealed that of all possible sources of information about how to succeed in clinical, the source that students trust *least* is the clinical instructor (Bowers, 1985). They believe that clinical instructors deliberately disguise their requirements and that it is not safe to inquire directly about any "hidden rules." This is a pedagogical example of the "hidden curriculum" and the "oppressed group behavior" that Terry Pitts and Joan Roberts have described in nursing.

By making the internal and often invisible external constraints explicit, critical theory attempts to create situations in which autonomous and responsible communication can occur. The goal of critical theory is to return systematically distorted communication to conditions of conversational rationality.

When discussing students' goals and assumptions, both teacher and student draw from a readily available stock of meanings. In other words, at any time in any community, there are certain salient or available vocabularies in which we voice our aspirations and explain our actions.

This pool of meanings or vocabulary is generated and reproduced by social mechanisms such as education and media. These are not democratically controlled or representative institutions (Giddens, 1979). Generations of research have demonstrated the domination of these institutions by certain class, race, and gender groups. Thus, meanings that favor the interests of these groups are more apt to survive and be reproduced than meanings that challenge their legitimacy or dominance (Shor, 1987; Popkewitz, 1984). We are all familiar with efforts to have more positive images of women and people of color inserted into the texts of media and education (Grumet, 1988).

Native speakers are often unaware of how their language has been shaped by the evolution of these institutions (Thompson, 1985, 1987). Yet, as we saw in the discussion of subjectivity, these vocabularies are not simply external to us, they become part of our identities. Our desires are socially produced within these vocabularies. Thus my language incorporates notions of masculinity that may prohibit my full achievement of my intimacy goals just as the woman's identity as patient and female blocked accomplishment of her health goals.

We developed an exercise to help nursing students become aware of their understandings of nursing and develop a basis for critiquing their views. In a large introduction to nursing class, we had students meet in small groups to articulate their definitions of a nurse-as-person and of nursing as an occupation. These definitions were synthesized into a collective list of attributes. Students then interviewed practicing nurses to ask them for their views of the nurse-as-person and nursing. Simultaneously they were reading Melosh's *Physician s Hand* and Reverby's *Ordered to Care* (Melosh, 1982; Reverby, 1987). In a series of writing and small group exercises, students first identified tensions and contradictions among the various views of nurses and nursing, used the historical texts to gain an understanding of the emergence of the language of nursing, and finally critiqued their initial definitions. Since I had these students again as seniors in a medical-surgical theory and clinical course, I had them revise and critique their assignments from the first course and explain what experiences they had had that led to a revision of their earlier views.

The purpose of these exercises was definitely not to develop "a" definition of nursing, but to gain an understanding of how these definitions change over time and often embody self-limiting meanings such as femininity and professionalism. Students also gained a perspective on how to open up such assumptions and revise their limitations.

Many examples of classroom practices such as this exist in the literature. Many more are used in classroom settings around the country by people like Barbara Hedin (1986), Peggy Chinn (Chinn & Wheeler, 1985), and Nancy Diekelmann. My interest lies not in highlighting my own teaching – which has been strongly influenced by these colleagues – but in stressing the complex interplay of understanding and emancipation within nursing discourse.

The revolutionary implications of critical social theory for educational practice are reflected in a dramatic reconceptualization of the nursing student as person. Once we acknowledge that science and education are grounded in contingent social agreement rather than ahistoric, transcendental, or universal principles, then we must attend to the communicative context in which science and education are negotiated. I firmly believe this means abandoning the moral wasteland of the technical perspective of students as raw material. In its place, we must commit to a vision of students as persons who enter nursing with traditions or horizons that motivate their projects of becoming nurses. We must understand the many types of nurses they envision, indeed, help them understand their own projects. At the same time, we must facilitate analysis of the systematic constraints that are embedded in their understandings. These constraints include contradictory and self-defeating vocabularies or discourses that have been shaped by domination and are structured into the communicative situation.

We can use this idea of contradictory and self-defeating vocabularies to clarify the relationship between critical social theory models of education – for example, that found in the writings of Paulo Freire – and feminist models. For the most part, Freire and other critical theorists such as Michael Apple (1982) have their origins in traditions that stress the differential interests of social classes in maintaining or revolutionizing educational practices. These theorists have not been clear enough about the intersection of class interests and gender interests (Weiler, 1988; Rosser, 1986). Given the gender composition of nursing and its location in male dominated administrative and medical networks, feminist analysis must give heightened attention to the contradictory and self-defeating languages that we all – male and female alike – bring into the classroom (Rothschild, 1988; Allen, 1986a).

We also have a responsibility to examine and critique our own understandings of nursing and nursing education. Conferences on the curriculum revolution are shining examples of our commitment to do so.

References

Allen, D. G. (1985). Nursing research and social control: Alternative models of science that emphasize understanding and emancipation. *Image: The Journal of Nursing Scholarship, 17*(2), 59-65.

Allen, D. G. (1986a). The use of philosophical and historical methodologies to understand the concept of "health." In P. L. Chinn (Ed.). *Nursing research methodology* (pp. 157-168). Rockville, MD: Aspen.

Allen, D. G. (1986b). Nursing and oppression: A feminist analysis of representations of "the family" in nursing textbooks. *Feminist Teacher, 2*(1), 15-20.

Allen, D. G. (1986c). Professionalism, gender segregation of labor and the control of nursing. *Women and Politics, 6*(3), 1-24.

Allen, D. G. (1987a). Critical social theory as a model for analyzing ethical issues in family and community health. *Family and Community Health, 10*(1), 63-72.

Allen, D. G. (1987b). The Social Policy Statement: A reappraisal. *Advances in Nursing Science, 10*(1), 39-48.

Allen, D. G., Allman, K., & Powers, P. (1990, May). *Feminist nursing research without gender.* Paper presented at Western Institute for Research in Nursing, Denver, CO.

Allen, D. G., Bowers, B., & Diekelmann, N. L. (1989). Writing to learn: A reconceptualization of thinking and writing in the nursing curriculum. *Journal of Nursing Education, 28*(1), 6-11.

Allen, D. G., & Wolfgram, B. (1988). Nursing, therapy and social control: Feminist science and systems-based family therapy. *Health Care for Women International, 9*, 107-124.

Apple, M. (1982). *Education and power.* Boston: Routledge & Kegan Paul.

Benhabib, S. (1986). *Critique, norm and utopia: A study of the foundations of critical theory.* New York: Columbia University Press.

Bernstein, R. (1983). *Beyond objectivism and relativism.* Philadelphia: University of Pennsylvania Press.

Bowers, B. (1985). *Students experience of undergraduate clinical.* San Francisco: Society for Research in Nursing Education.

Chinn, P. L., & Wheeler, C. (1985). Feminism and nursing. *Nursing Outlook, 33*(2), 74-77.

Culley, M., & Portuges, C. (1985). *Gendered subjects: The dynamics of feminist teaching.* Boston: Routledge & Kegan Paul.

Diekelmann, N. L. (1990). Nursing education: Caring, dialogue and practice. *Journal of Nursing Education, 29*(7), 300-306.

Diekelmann, N. L., Allen, D. G., & Tanner, C. A. (1989). *The NLN criteria for appraisal of baccalaureate programs: A critical hermeneutic analysis.* New York: National League for Nursing.

Freire, P. (1986). *Pedagogy of the oppressed.* New York: Continuum.

Freire, P. (1987). *Education for critical consciousness.* New York: Continuum.

Giddens, A. (1979). *Central problems in social theory.* London: Macmillan.

Giroux, H. (1988). *Teachers as intellectuals.* Boston: Bergin & Garvey.

Grumet, M. (1988). *Bitter milk: Women and teaching.* Amherst: University of Massachusetts Press.

Habermas, J. (1979). *Knowledge and human interests* (J. Shapiro, Trans.). Boston: Beacon. (Original work published 1968)

Habermas, J. (1984). *The theory of communicative action: Volume 1, Reason and the rationalization of society* (T. McCarthy, Trans.). Boston: Beacon. (Original work published 1981)

Habermas, J. (1987). *The theory of communicative action: Volume 2, Life world and system* (T. McCarthy, Trans.). Boston: Beacon.

Harding, S. (1986). *The science question in feminism.* Ithaca, NY: Cornell University Press.

Hedin, B. (1986). A case study of oppressed group behavior in nurses. *Image: The Journal of Nursing Scholarship, 18*(2), 53-57.

Kuhn, T. (1962). *The structure of scientific revolutions.* Chicago: University of Chicago Press.

Melosh, B. (1982). *The physician s hand.* Philadelphia: Temple University Press.

Misgeld, D. (1985). Education and cultural invasion: Critical social theory, education as instruction, and the pedagogy of the oppressed. In J. Forester (Ed.). *Critical theory and public life* (pp. 77-120). Cambridge, MA: MIT Press.

Nicholson, C. (1989). Postmodernism, feminism, and education: The need for solidarity. *Educational Theory, 39*(3), 197-205.

Pagano, J. A. (1988). Teaching women. *Educational Theory, 38*(3), 321-339.

Pitts, T. P. (1985). The covert curriculum: What does nursing education really teach? *Nursing Outlook, 33*(1), 37-42.

Popkewitz, T. (1984). *Paradigm and ideology in educational research.* New York: Falmer.

Reverby, S. (1987). *Ordered to care: The dilemma of American nursing, 1850 1945.* New York: Cambridge University Press.

Roberts, S. (1983). Oppressed group behavior: Implications for nursing. *Advances in Nursing Science, 5*(4), 21-30.

Rose, H. (1983). Hand, brain and heart: A feminist epistemology for the natural sciences. *Signs, 9*(1), 73-90.

Rosser, S. (1986). *Teaching science and health from a feminist perspective.* New York: Pergamon.

Rothschild, J. (1988). *Teaching technology from a feminist perspective.* New York: Pergamon.

Shor, I. (1987). *Critical teaching and everyday life.* Chicago: University of Chicago Press.

Thompson, J. (1985). Practical discourse in nursing: Going beyond empiricism and historicism. *Advances in Nursing Science, 7*(4), 59-71.

Thompson, J. (1987). Critical scholarship: The critique of domination in nursing. *Advances in Nursing Science, 10*(1), 27-38.

Thompson, J. (1990). Hermeneutic inquiry. In L. Moody (Ed.). *Advancing nursing science through research,* Vol II. Newbury Park: Sage.

Weiler, K. (1988). *Women teaching for change: Gender, class and power.* Boston: Bergin & Garvey.

White, S. (1988). *The recent work of Jürgen Habermas: Reason, justice and modernity.* New York: Cambridge University Press.

A Response to David Allen: Critical Social Theory and Nursing Education

Jane Sumner

David Allen's (1990) chapter on critical social theory (CST) and nursing education remains as important as when first written. Unfortunately, this philosophical perspective has not been pursued as it might have been. The implications of this failure are of concern in an era of rapidly changing health care delivery, and nurses' roles and functions within it. If nursing education is the first step into professional nursing practice, then it is relevant that the critical social theory lens be applied to how we nurse educators think about our educational models and what needs to be changed. Why? Because it forces one to confront comfortable but infrequently challenged daily norms. Are our customary ways of educating student nurses really producing nurses who are ready practice in the "Brave New World?"

Porter-O'Grady (2001) has challenged nurse educators to prepare students to be creative, flexible, adaptable, and capable of analytical and critical thinking in any health care delivery situation, and as nurse educators we must ask ourselves if we are in fact achieving this. Or are we still "training" students rather than creating environments where students are learners and are stimulated to learn and to think? Allen disparages the "training" of skills, but I would make a strong counter-argument that these skills are part of the social communication between nurses and patients and remain important. I would agree, however that "training" is insufficient. Are we producing registered nurses who may not be ready to practice in the current shifting sands of the health care delivery system?

Do our educational models acknowledge that health care delivery in the United States is white, middle class and empiricist, yet US society is very different from that? In addition, the human condition is much more complicated, less rational and more complex than detached scientific objectivity generally acknowledges. Neither nurses nor patients necessarily "fit" this particular construct of the health care system, yet both are expected to conform within it.

Allen claimed that CST is a philosophy rather than a method; however, more recent authors (Althiede & Johnson, 1994; Alvesson & Sköldberg, 2000; Kincheloe & McLaren, 2003) suggest that it provides a lens through which one can examine unquestioned norms and shibboleths. They suggest that CST as method is a very useful contribution in qualitative research. The goal of critical social theory as a method of analysis is to try to understand both the historical context and the current (or modern) social context. The concern is "consciousness, subjectivity, culture, ideology…in order to make possible…change" (Kellner, 1989, p. 12). Allen (1995) indicated some of the foundational assumptions of nursing are embedded in the traditional role of women and medical paternalism, which has historically "systematically devalued" (1995, p. 176) the nursing profession. These assumptions need careful scrutiny in today's context of the health care delivery system. Historic, organizational, political, and economic factors create a power hierarchy which can manipulate communication, and as a result the symbols of language are distorted (Campbell & Bunting, 1991; Kellner, 1989). A critical social theory perspective forces examination of power and its use and/or manipulation. Do we as nurse educators unconsciously wield power over our students that does not facilitate learning? In addition, we, as nurse educators, must ask ourselves about our nursing symbols that we hold most dear: whether they are appropriate for today's practice world, and whether they are universals.

Where do nursing and nurses fit into the power hierarchy of the "governmentality" that is the "matrices of power as surveillance" (Cheek, 2000, p. 27) of health care delivery systems' bureaucracies? What is autonomy, and is there autonomy for nurses? Nurse educators talk about it and indicate that to be genuine patient advocates we must be autonomous. What is the real meaning of the symbol "autonomy" for nursing? Does this mean power?

Has art knowledge been so distorted that it has been marginalized and devalued? Has science knowledge emerged as the dominant power? Utilizing a CST lens facilitates exploration of the dichotomy between art knowledge and science knowledge in nursing as a critique of power. Madeleine Leininger as early as the 1960s was beginning to ask about the influence of the "medicalization" of nursing (1991). Her perspective was through a caring lens, but her points are well taken if nursing is regarded as the skilled and knowledgeable care and comfort offered the human condition, and this is far more inclusive than illness/treatment or cure, our present-time focus. Have nurse educators become so enraptured with the science or "medicalization" of nursing that they have forgotten the caring mandate of the profession? The caring mandate is not merely for illness, but for the whole person who is the patient.

As nursing education has become more driven by Tylerian behavioral outcomes and the "science" of nursing, one must ask what has been lost overall? How have these perspectives been colored by the medicalization of nursing? Has there perhaps been an overemphasis on the science of nursing? These issues must be seen through the prism of efforts to claim nursing as a "profession." Strenuous efforts were being made to oust nursing from under the paternalistic control of medicine, which included shifting nursing education out of hospitals into universities, making claims for both autonomy and responsibility, and increasingly today being pressured by the demand for evidence-based nursing practice. What seems to have been slipping away is any emphasis on the highly skilled art of comfort and concern for the individual human being. In addition, there is a danger that the human needs of nurses are being lost or overlooked, and this is worrisome.

Critical social theory is the critique of hegemonic power, which "question[s] the framework of the way we organize our lives or the ways our lives are organized for us, it probes foundational assumptions that are normally taken for granted" (Foster, 1986, p. 72). A critical social theory lens aids in interpreting and evaluating professional caring in nursing in ways that can liberate the profession from paternalistic control. Not only can a CST perspective be applied to organizations and relationships between people, it can also stimulate critical reflection into self, which can be enlightening, empowering, emancipating, and lead to reframed perception, thinking, and action (Henderson, 1995; Johns, 1995). There is a powerful argument that this should be an emphasis of nursing education. Particularly if nurses are to practice autonomously, and understand themselves and how they use themselves in practice, then critical self-reflection is crucial.

Alvesson and Sköldberg (2000) described CST research as "triple hermeneutics" (p. 144). The first stage is an individual's interpretation of him/herself and his/her subjective reality and its meaning to him/her. The second stage is the researcher's interpretation of this reality. The third stage is the "critical interpretation of unconscious processes, ideologies, power relations, and other expressions of dominance that entail the privilege of certain interests over others, within the forms of understanding which appear to be spontaneously generated" (p. 144). It is this third stage that is the most difficult for a researcher, because one is acculturated into an ethos of particular values and norms. It is not easy to distance oneself from these familiar, largely unquestioned narratives. As a method, CST stimulates the following questions: What are the false assumptions? Where and what are the gaps and silences? Is there anything wrong with the accepted norms? What are the historical constraints and implications for nursing practice today?

Allen took advantage of Jürgen Habermas' (1979, 1984, 1987) theories on "social rationality," with its technical, practical, and emancipatory interests and discussed these within the context of nursing education. Habermas belonged to the Frankfurt School of Critical Theory, and if one is interested in the philosopher, then one becomes curious about critical social theory. Habermas' early work was Marxist, which in itself has been criticized and critiqued; however, with time he moved away from the political implications of Marxism and became more philosophical in trying to understand the human condition. I would aver that this is why he is of interest to nurses who are trying to understand nursing. What Allen did not discuss was Habermas' later Theory of Communicative Action and Moral Consciousness (1992), which elucidates his earlier work, and I believe is highly relevant and important for nursing in its specific social life-world. I was drawn to Allen's thinking because I too felt Jürgen Habermas' philosophy offered some different ways of thinking about nursing and its various contexts, but also because of Habermas' fundamental understanding of the universalities of the human condition. He recognizes that humans are social beings who interact only through discourse and this makes the individual open and vulnerable.

It is the later work that caught my interest and led to my own theory development, and its subsequent application to nursing education. Habermas merged the three interests into his communicative action and moral consciousness theory. But it was his premise of moral consciousness that distilled my thinking about nursing, nurses, patients, and the communication that is the essence of the relationship. He wrote about individuals only being able to mature through socialization or communication, but this left them open and vulnerable. It is the latter that demands "considerateness" (Habermas, 1992, p. 198), and it is this that is the moral component of his thinking. For me, that was simple in relation to patients, but I quickly realized that it applied to all humans, and thus the nurse too. From there it was relatively straightforward. I was able to separate the nurse into the personal and professional self, the latter having three knowledges, theory, practice, and experiential, and the patient who is both a personal and illness self. The third component was the communication between them. Habermas discussed three claims to normative validity: the claim to truth (or factual rational knowledge), the claim to truthfulness (the intrasubjective self) and the claim to right (intersubjective world). I have been able to utilize these claims in my own theory (Sumner, 2000, 2001). It makes sense to me. Nursing is practiced in an intimate life-world of intersubjective connections in which each is in need of considerateness. I make the argument that Habermas' three levels of moral maturity, preconventional, conventional and postconventional, also can be applied to the nurse-patient relationship, although whether the highest level can be achieved by the patient is debatable and may be difficult for any but the most seasoned nurse. But the reality of human vulnerability with the need for considerateness for both nurse and patient is the central concept of my own work and I would strongly argue is valid in the communication of the specialized life-world of the health care delivery systems.

Bishop and Scudder (1990) discussed Triadic Dialogue in which they clearly separate the patient self from the illness, and they state there are two subjects and one object in any discourse. In this instance, the object is the illness, and the patient and nurse are both speaker and listener, focusing on the illness, which is a separate entity. This added to my work, because it ensured that the patient remained human and was not objectified. From Bishop and Scudder's Triadic Dialogue and my own thinking I have been able to develop an educational model, "Quadrangular Dialogue" (2004), in which the players are nurse educator, nursing student, patient and it is the illness that is the object for the three humans, who are all subjects.

My perspective is that CST facilitates deep reflection, which I think is critical to optimize student learning, but also for maximum patient outcomes and growth in the nurse educator. This approach also stimulates examination of the power structure in the nurse educator-student relationship, the student-patient relationship, and the nurse educator-student-patient relationship. In addition to the intersubjective and intrasubjective possibilities offered by a CST lens, there is an opportunity to examine the power structure of the school and the potential for coercive and bullying behaviors within the organization.

Taking advantage of Habermas' theory means that the vulnerabilities of all the humans in the school and clinical settings are acknowledged, which means that discourse is facilitated where all the voices are heard. The communication is between equal human beings. The knowledge and skill development is not ignored in this model; rather, they are thoughtfully encouraged by the nurse educator for the student to think about and learn. A CST approach means one can continually ask questions about what is missing and how the education model will enable the student to graduate with the skills that Porter-O'Grady (2001) indicated were essential for today's practicing professional nurse. We as a profession and as nurse educators have need for ongoing research utilizing CST methodology in order to shape curricula that will meet Porter-O'Grady's challenge.

David Allen's thoughtful chapter is truly relevant and continues to be important today, although his gap lies in that he did not have available to him Habermas' later work where the technical, emancipatory, and practical interests are further developed in the normative claims to validity. It is the understanding of moral consciousness in relation to the vulnerability of the human condition and the need for considerateness that has particular relevance for nursing and nursing education. Nevertheless, Allen's observations on curriculum, the student, and the nurse educator remain valid today.

References

Allen, D. G. (1995). Hermeneutics: Philosophical traditions and nursing practice research. *Nursing Science Quarterly, 8*(4), 174-182.

Altheide, D. L., & Johnson, J. M. (1994). Criteria for assessing interpretive validity in qualitative research. In N. K. Denzin, & Y. S. Lincoln (Eds.). *Handbook of qualitative research*. Thousand Oaks, CA: Sage.

Alvesson, M. & Sköldberg, K. (2000). *Reflexive methodology: New vistas for qualitative research*. Thousand Oaks, CA: Sage.

Bishop, A. H., & Scudder, J. R. (1990). *The practical, moral, and personal sense of nursing*. New York: State University of New York Press.

Campbell, J. C., & Bunting, S. (1991). Voices and paradigms: Perspectives on critical and feminist theory in nursing. *Advances in Nursing Science, 13*(3), 1-15.

Cheek, J. (2000). *Postmodern and poststructural approaches to nursing research*. Thousand Oaks, CA: Sage.

Foster, W. (1986). *Paradigms and promises*. Amherst, NY: Prometheus Books.

Habermas, J. (1979). *Knowledge and human interests* (J. Shapiro, Trans.). Boston: Beacon. (Original work published 1968)

Habermas, J. (1984). *The theory of communicative action: Volume 1, Reason and the rationalization of society* (T. McCarthy, Trans.). Boston: Beacon. (Original work published 1981)

Habermas, J. (1987). *The theory of communicative action: Volume 2, Life world and system* (T. McCarthy, Trans.). Boston: Beacon.

Habermas, J. (1992). *Moral consciousness and communicative action* (C. Lenhardt & S. W. Nicholsen, Trans.). Cambridge, MA: MIT Press. (Original work published 1983)

Henderson, D. J. (1995). Consciousness raising in participatory research: Method and methodology for emancipatory inquiry. *Advances in Nursing Science, 17*(3), 58-69.

Johns, C. (1995). Framing learning through reflection within Carper's fundamental ways of knowing in nursing. *Journal of Advanced Nursing, 22*, 226-234.

Kellner, D. (1989). *Critical theory, Marxism, and modernity.* Baltimore: Johns Hopkins University Press.

Kincheloe, J. L., & McLaren, P. L. (2003). Rethinking critical theory and qualitative research. In N. K. Denzin, & Y. S. Lincoln (Eds.). *The landscape of qualitative research: Theories and issues.* Thousand Oaks, CA: Sage.

Leininger, M. M. (1991). *Culture care diversity & universality: A theory of nursing.* New York: National League for Nursing Press.

Porter-O'Grady, T. (2001). Profound change: 21st century nurse. *Nursing Outlook, 49*, 182-186.

Sumner, J. (2000). *Caring in nursing: A critical theory study.* Unpublished dissertation. University of New Orleans, New Orleans, LA.

Sumner, J. (2001). Caring in nursing: A different interpretation. *Journal of Advanced Nursing, 35*, 926-932.

Sumner, J. (2004). Case study: Quadrangular Dialogue: A caring in nursing teaching model. *International Journal of Nursing Education Scholarship,* 1(1), Article 7. http://www.bepress.com/ijnes/vol1/iss1/art7.

Feminist Pedagogy in Nursing Education[1]

Peggy L. Chinn

Pedagogy is the art, science, or profession of teaching. Pedagogy, as an idea, is as old as education itself. However, those who teach and those who learn are most often unaware of what constitutes the particular pedagogy with which they are working.

Pedagogy Within a Patriarchy

Pedagogy is something that is alive; it is a total package. It exists in the actions we take in the learning environment, the materials we use, how we use them, and the attitudes we convey. All teaching and learning encounters can be characterized by pedagogy. Most pedagogies we use today are patriarchal or masculinist, in that they derive from ideas about how to teach and learn that come from a predominantly male experience of the world. The content that is identified as important to learn comes from the same source. The "authorities" and authoritative literature from whom we glean the specific content to be learned is almost always that of male authors, derived from male experience and views of the world. The skills that are thought of as useful to learn are identified because of their ultimate value in male-dominated social and political systems. The attitudes that are thought of as important to instill in students are identified as valuable for learning because they are the attitudes that serve us well in male-defined situations. The "logic" that is thought to characterize the educated mind is a logic of masculinist thinking.

The institutions in which we do our teaching are patriarchal institutions, arranged in power-over hierarchies that diminish human experience, despite the educational philosophies of important humanist forefathers. The language that is used to describe existing pedagogies reflects assumptions and views of the world that derive from patriarchal ideologies and world views, which are seldom questioned (Spender, 1982). Consider examples such as:

- *Grades.* Alphabetical characters that are assigned a rank order and given numerical value that is multiplied and divided at will, and used for purposes of life-shattering consequence. One wonders, grades of what, for what end? Who benefits?

- *Teacher student.* The "one" who knows and gives, the "other" who does not know and absorbs that which is given, preferably without questioning. Both are usually assumed to be male unless proven otherwise.

- *Lecture.* A one-way communication of pouring forth, declaring "truth"; the ultimate in expression of the syndrome "academentia" (Daly & Caputi, 1987). Usually based on knowledge set forth by male "authority" regardless of the gender of the lecturer.

1. Originally published in *Curriculum revolution: Reconceptualizing nursing education* (1989, pp. 9-24). New York: National League for Nursing. Reprinted with permission.

- *Course.* The one appropriate path to knowledge, prescribed by institutions that charge a fee for taking the path, and measured in numbers of hours spent sitting in a specified room, in a specified chair.

- *Objectives.* The ultimate tautology – objectives are defined by the teacher, the giver of knowledge, as that which is worthy to know and learn, and it is the teacher who declares their achievement. This concept was conceived by male victims of logical thought. Usually achievement of these linguistic descriptors is measured by numerical signifiers, usually in examinations.

- *Examinations.* The "one" who truly "knows" places the "other" in a particularly uncomfortable and threatening situation, which is deemed all the better to "prove" whether the other "knows" anything at all.

Given these realities, a shift to feminist pedagogy is a radical shift. Pedagogically, there is nothing that can be taken for granted. Everything we do in preparing for the learning encounter, the content we plan, the language we use, the way we conduct ourselves, what we value, the attitudes we convey, the behaviors we nurture, the literature we draw on, the way we think about our purpose, what we hope to accomplish – everything – takes a dramatic shift into an entirely different realm (Weiler, 1988). For feminism itself is a dramatic shift in relation to the world as we now know it and experience it.

Feminism is valuing women, and all that is associated in our culture with women and women's experience. Feminist pedagogy derives from content that is viewed and experienced with women at the center. It draws on women's writings and other forms of women's accounts of their views and experience. (Note that women have been excluded from literary circles for centuries; therefore our literature is not limited to what is typically thought of as "literature.") It draws on skills that are central to women's experience. It nurtures attitudes that are valued in terms of women's realities. It draws on women's ways of thinking.

Feminist pedagogy can sometimes be seen as being in a dialectic relationship with masculinist pedagogy, but in my opinion, the two are not in a strictly dialectic posture with one another. Masculinist ideas and pedagogies have existed for centuries without a glimmer of concern for women's experience, realities, or views, even though they have been sustained and made possible by the material energy, scrubbing, feeding, and nurturing of countless women. Feminist ideas derive, in large part, from this very experience of supporting and making possible the masculinist world of reality. Therefore, a feminist view takes that reality into account. (Feminist ideas consistently flow in a direction of healing splits in our experience and in our thinking, seeking to bring together that which can be, with that which is.) Feminist methods are based on the premise that perceiving the whole leads to a fuller and richer understanding of what we know, and how we know it.

Sandra Harding (1987) has pointed out that a feminist standpoint is not something anyone can have by claiming it, but an achievement. (A standpoint differs in this respect from a perspective.) To achieve a feminist standpoint one must engage in the intellectual and political struggle necessary to see nature and social life from the point of view of that disdained activity which produces women's social experiences instead of from the partial and perverse perspective available from the "ruling gender" experience of men (p. 185).

This insight explains how feminist ideas can develop within the context of patriarchal institutions like schools and universities, and how we as teachers can do the political work of feminist pedagogy within those walls. As we do so, we experience the material realities of the intellectual and political struggle that are essential to achieving a feminist standpoint. We begin to consciously do what we know. As we act, we learn about a new way of being in the world.

Pedagogy, Feminism, and Nursing

This is an extremely important undertaking for women who are nurses. The two ideas – pedagogy and feminism – have profound, indeed radical, meaning for nursing education. When we bring these two ideas together, we have a profound shift in the highly political process of education. In the context of nursing education, we begin to create a foundation for a profound shift in health care.

We begin to assume a questioning, skeptical stance toward everything that we have previously thought and known, and we become open to possibilities that we had never before taken seriously. The experience is transformative; it begins within. The shifts are both familiar and strange. Most of what we begin to experience are ways of being and doing that are familiar to everyone, particularly to women. However, at the same time they also feel strange because they are ways of thinking and being that have for our entire lives been devalued; and that we have worked to deny, compartmentalize, or see as somehow less than useful. These ways of thinking and doing do not exclude some of the possibilities that predominate in the masculinist world, which is why I sometimes find a dialectic view of these pedagogies to be less than useful. Rather, all possibilities are considered and questioned, but what remains constant is the fundamental commitment in relation to women and women's experience, and an ethic based on this perspective.

Pedagogy, Praxis, and Power

Feminist pedagogy is based on a feminist praxis. Feminist praxis incorporates thoughtful reflection and action that occur in synchrony toward the goal of transforming the world. The transformation that is sought is a vision that is grounded in feminist ethics and ideas about the way the world could be for all people. Central to feminist visions about the world as it could be is consciousness – full awareness that is based on a conviction that "I Know what I Do, and I Do what I Know" (Wheeler & Chinn, 1989).

Feminist praxis is concerned with power. Feminist praxis consciously rejects "power over" forms of power, but rather seeks personal empowerment and exercise of personal power in the world that leads to growth, transformation, unity, justice, and peace. How women experience power in our own lives (our own power or lack of it, or the powers of others over us) is central to the conceptions that have developed about power from a feminist perspective.

Power, and the closely related concept of empowerment, is therefore central to feminist pedagogy. Charlene Wheeler and I have conceptualized feminist forms of power in relation to group process and in relation to a teaching-learning experience. These feminist forms of power are derived from a perspective that values women and women's realities, along with women's concerns about how the world could be. These powers and some specific ways in which they are enacted in teaching and learning are:

Power of Process

Objectives, time frames, and educational structures of evaluation may be used as tools that provide a structure from which to work, but they are not the focal point. The *process* is the important dimension, so that once the interaction begins, the structure is *only* a tool and nothing more. *How* the interactions happen become the central focus, rather than a precise adherence to a prescribed content. Language is chosen as a tool to make the process possible, to create mental images that reduce the power imbalances of the institution and create new relationships. The process itself becomes part of the "text" for teaching and learning.

Power of Letting Go

All participants let go of old habits and ways in order to make room for personal and collective growth. Teachers let go of "power over" attitudes and ways of being; registrants let go of "tell me what to do" attitudes and ways of being. All participants move into ways of being that are personally empowering and that also nurture the empowerment of others.

Power of the Whole

Mutual help networks within the group are encouraged. Every individual is responsible to invest talents and skills for the interests of the group as a whole. Each participant, whether teacher or registrant, is accountable to the whole group for negotiating specific agendas, keeping the group informed as to absences, leaving early, arriving late, or initiating particular learning experiences.

Power of Collectivity

Each participant is taken into account in the group's planning-in-process. The group works to address the needs of learners who are moving into individual journeys where others may not be going. The needs of learners who are having specific struggles are addressed by the group in some way. Learners do not compete with one another; rather, the needs of all learners are acknowledged and addressed as equally valuable.

Power of Unity

Unity is viewed as coming from the expression of conflict and differing points of view so that the various points of view can be understood by all, and integrated into a richer and fuller appreciation of every individual. Learning is not merely accumulating the truths that are passed along by an authority, or accepting those ideas as "truth," but rather is an attitude of actively seeking to understand the possibilities of differing perspectives.

Power of Sharing

All participants enter the group with talents, skills, and abilities related to the education project, and actively engage in sharing their individual talents with the group. Teachers enter learning groups with previously developed capabilities that are shared according to the needs of the group and in consideration of the structure-as-tool. Registrants enter the group with personal talents, backgrounds, and experiences that are valued and shared. All participants enter the group as learners, open to what others can share.

Power of Integration

All dimensions of the situation are acknowledged to form a whole experience. Each individual's unique and self-defined needs for the learning experience are acknowledged and integrated into the process. The first portion of each gathering is used as a time for each individual to express her or his priorities, needs, and wishes for the gathering so that these can be integrated as a part of the process for that gathering.

Power of Nurturing

Each participant is respected fully and unconditionally, and treated as necessary and integral to the experience of the group. Learning activities and approaches are planned to nurture the gradual growth of new skills and abilities, assuring that every participant can be successful both in terms of the planned structure of the experience, and in terms of her or his individual needs.

Power of Intuition

The process that occurs, and the nature of what is addressed in the learning encounter depend as much on the experience of the moment as on any other factor. What emerges as important for the group to address in the moment is what happens. Letting go of what "ought" to happen is valued as a new skill that makes possible what will happen.

Power of Consciousness

Ethical dimensions of the process, as well as the content of the learning experience, are central for reaching heightened awareness. A portion of each gathering, usually toward the end, is devoted to a closing "ritual" that includes criticism, where everyone reflects on the process of the gathering, what it meant, and ways in which the intended values were enacted.

Power of Diversity

Deliberate processes are planned and enacted to integrate points of view of individuals and groups whose perspectives are usually not addressed. The experiences (through writings, personal encounters, poetry, song, drama, etc.) of minority groups, of different classes, of third-world people, of women, are given a deliberate focus during the learning experience. In nursing education, nursing itself has been so long devalued as an important resource for learning, that it represents a diversity apart from the mainstream of the health care system. Thus, nursing literature, experience, stories, and ways of knowing are consciously emphasized.

Power of Responsibility

All participants assume full responsibility as the agent for her or his role in the process. The experience is planned to provide some structure that assures every participant the opportunity to assume a leadership role during the experience. "Grades" are viewed as each individual's responsibility; they are viewed as a tool to represent what the individual earns through demonstrated accomplishments. Teachers assume responsibility to demystify the processes involved in all planned activities, including provisions for evaluation and grades and other expectations imposed by the structure of the institution.

Practical Suggestions for Using a Feminist Pedagogy

There are many ways in which the feminist concepts of power can be enacted in a learning situation. The suggestions here are certainly not the only way; they are examples taken from my own experience. I have used the approaches described here with groups of 6 to 40 students.

The size of the groups in which the process has been most successful is about 20. Traditional pedagogies do not provide a means for everyone present to fully participate, and the shift that makes this possible begins to be most apparent in this size group.

In order to demystify all elements of the experience, I have used the course syllabus as a means of providing detailed information about the pedagogical premises and methods, as well as guidelines for the gatherings that are appropriate to the course content. I have included the structure of the curriculum: course description, objectives, and listings of texts. I have used *Peace & Power: A Handbook of Feminist Process* (Wheeler & Chinn, 1984, 1989) as a reading the first week after the group convenes as a means of introducing everyone to the group process that we will use.

The syllabus contains four major elements: philosophy of the course design, a description of the learning activities that are planned as a structure from which we can work, the suggested provisions for how each participant can earn a grade that demonstrates her or his competence, and a working outline from which the group can plan each gathering. The following sections provide examples taken from the syllabus of a first semester graduate course on nursing theory development.

Example of the "Philosophy of the Course Design"

The activities and interactions in this course are planned to enact the philosophy of the School of Nursing, and the philosophic basis upon which nursing theory is developed.

The emphasis is on:

- Creativity

- Humanistic care

- The autonomy and unique individuality of each participant

- The growth and development of all participants

All participants have different and unique experiences and talents; all are valued equally. In order for the ideal of equal participation and valuing to be actualized, all participants assume full responsibility and accountability. It is the responsibility of all participants to actively value their own, and each other participant's, critical thought, experiences, knowledge, and talents.

The faculty role in this experience is based on the desire to eliminate the unequal power relationships that exist within current institutionalized educational settings. The faculty is a participant and a learner along with all other participants, not the expert, judge, or "guru." The faculty enters with experience and background in relation to the focus of the course, and is responsible for preparing materials that can be used as a starting point for learning and development, providing resources for planning each discussion with the co-conveners, and for providing feedback and constructive criticism for all activities designed to demonstrate competence in relation to learning.

The faculty is obligated to provide evidence of each individual's completion of the learning objectives in the form of a grade. However, the grade for the course is earned, not given. The faculty participates with each individual in assessing work that demonstrates the grade that is earned.

Example of "Learning Activities"

1. Discussion Convening. At least once, each participant will work with another participant to convene the gathering. This requires in-depth reading of all the

planned readings for the gathering, and meeting with faculty and/or co-convener(s) before the gathering to plan the agenda. Individuals volunteer for convening responsibilities at least one week in advance. Convening provides the opportunity to practice leadership in a safe environment, where group feedback and support can be provided.

2. Reading and Participation in Discussion. For each gathering there are planned readings; these and any other readings you select provide a basis for active discussion. Discussions also draw on personal experiences, so your personal journal (described below) will be important to help you reflect on the meaning of this experience.

There are several short stories on reserve in the library that are planned for reading within the first four weeks of the semester. The purposes of the short stories are to provide: 1) a common "clinical experience" for discussing the practice implications of theoretical ideas, 2) insight and inspiration in creative expression, and 3) experience related to the esthetic pattern of knowing in nursing.

Being Present (in mind, body, and spirit) is important both for individual learning and for the development of the group as a whole. During check-in, each participant connects with the group and uses this sharing to help everyone integrate individual needs and agendas for the gathering. If an individual must be absent, leave early or otherwise interrupt the discussion, that individual lets everyone in the group know in advance so all can anticipate and plan for the shift in group dynamics.

Each discussion will conclude with appreciation, criticism, and affirmation. During this time each person reflects on the process of the gathering, the extent to which the group process facilitated individual and group development, and explores suggestions for moving ahead.

3. Personal Journal. All participants keep a personal journal or diary throughout the semester. The journal provides a record of your personal growth and development, and can serve as the basis for other learning activities such as group discussions or writing. The journal is not shared, except in rare instances. The central purpose of the journal is to explore avenues of personal knowing in nursing.

4. Scholarly Writing. A scholarly paper related to the learning objectives of the course is planned as the primary avenue for demonstrating your accomplishments. The primary purpose of the writing is to explore the potential for development of nursing knowledge. At least two drafts of the writing will be shared. One copy of each draft is shared with faculty and one copy with another participant. Reviewers provide constructive criticism in the interest of helping you develop your ideas. A suggested schedule for assuring completion of the writing during the semester is included in the detailed topical outline for the semester.

5. Critique of Colleague's Writing. Each participant will review a colleague's first draft of the written work and write a brief summary of suggestions and comments. These will be shared with the author to use as needed; a copy of the review will be provided for the faculty, to document your participation in this activity, and for faculty feedback to help develop this skill.

Example of "Grading" Proposal

Grading. All participants earn a grade of "B" on completion of the following:

- *Co convenes* group discussions as needed to provide leadership for all the gatherings. Each participant will co-convene at least once; if the group is small, additional responsibilities for co-convening will be mutually agreed upon by the group. The quality of convening will be reflected in the criticism/self-criticism portion of the discussion; the grade is not affected.

- *Participates actively in discussion* during each gathering, with no more than three absences during the semester, unless negotiated differently with the entire group.

- *Provides written criticism* of a colleague's early draft(s) of written work. Copies of an adapted ANS (*Advances in Nursing Science*) review form are provided to facilitate developing skills of constructive criticism. The review is shared with the author of the paper, and with the faculty as evidence of completion and competence in written criticism. Reviews are not "graded" nor will they affect the grade of the author of the written work that is reviewed.

- *Prepares a scholarly essay* that is shared with faculty and with another participant in the group in draft and final forms. Every reviewer provides constructive criticism of the work-in-progress to aid the author in developing the essay. The faculty is responsible for assessing the work in relation to the grade, and will discuss with the author any concerns related to the grade the individual is earning. The criteria on which a grade of "B" is based are provided on the adapted *Advances in Nursing Science* review form as follows:

    I. Consistency with the course objectives.

    II. Concise, logical ordering of ideas; readability.

    III. Sound argument and defense of original ideas.

    IV. Accuracy of content.

    V. Appropriate use of methods of scholarly investigation.

    VI. Adequacy of documentation.

"A" Grade. An "A" grade is earned by demonstrating excellence. An "A" grade is earned by individuals who:

- Demonstrate competence in all planned learning activities.

- Participate actively in all gatherings, with no more than one absence during the semester.

- Share an enrichment project with the group that is contracted with the group as a whole. The group is responsible for agreeing that the project is related to our mutual goals and that it will provide enrichment for the individual and for the group.

"C" Grade or lower. The processes of the course are designed to provide maximum opportunity for early, open feedback, discussion, and negotiation along the way to assure that each participant earns the grade that is sought. A grade of "C" or lower will be recorded if these processes are not successful.

Incomplete grade. Incompletes will not be used for this course; if you begin to have problems in completing the learning activities, you are urged to consult with faculty as early as possible, and to withdraw from the course.

Examples from Detailed "Topical Outline"

The following are extracts from a complete topical outline. These extracts illustrate the planning for a gradual development of writing skills and learning the skills of providing constructive critique of a colleague's writing. The suggested readings illustrate the integration of a diversity of "voices" and avenues for introducing a perspective based on women's experiences of the world.

WEEK #2
DEVELOPMENT OF KNOWLEDGE (SEPTEMBER 19)
(Course Objectives: 1.1, 1.2, 1.3)

Conveners:_____

Readings:

Phillips, D. C. (1987). *Philosophy, science and social inquiry* (Part A: Expositions: Recent philosophical developments, pp. 2-45). New York: Pergamon.

Spender, D. (1982). *Invisible women: The schooling scandal* (Introduction, Chapters 1 & 2, pp. 1-38). London: Writers and Readers Publishing Cooperative.

Wheeler, C. E., & Chinn, P. L. (1985). *Peace and power: A handbook of feminist process.* Buffalo: Margaretdaughters.

Woolf, V. (1979). Women and fiction. In M. Barrett (Ed.), *Virginia Woolf: Women and writing* (pp. 43-52). New York: Harcourt Brace Jovanovich. (Reprinted from The Forum, 1929).

Selected Short Stories. The stories that are on reserve include:

Browne, Susan E.: "Infusing Blues." True story of a nurse with diabetes and her struggle in gaining control. (biographical)

Finger, Annie: "Like the Hully Gully but Not So Slow." True story of a teenager with physical disability and her conflicts with her family. (biographical)

Geller, Ruth: "The Island." Story of a nurse dealing with the stress of her work/personal life. (fiction)

Geller, Ruth: "The Woman with My Eyes." Story involving a patient from Buffalo Psych Center and a worker in the experimental laboratory. (fiction)

Gilman, Charlotte Perkins: "The Yellow Wallpaper." Story of postpartum depression. (partly autobiographical, partly fiction)

LeGuin, Ursula K.: "Mazes." Story involving scientific experimentation. (fiction)

O'Connor, Flannery: "The Geranium." Story of an old man's day-to-day survival. (fiction)

Olsen, Tillie: "I Stand Here Ironing." Story involving a mother's reflections on raising her troubled daughter. (fiction)

Rose, Susan: "Pictures from a Family Album." Story told in the voice of an abused child. (fiction)

Learning Activities:

Begin personal journal.

Suggestion: Reflect on the meaning of the readings to you. Write about experiences and events that remind you of readings this week.

WEEK #3

PHILOSOPHY AND HISTORY OF NURSING SCIENCE (SEPTEMBER 26)

(Course Objectives 3.1, 3.3)

Conveners:_____

Readings:

Carper, B. (1987, October). Fundamental patterns of knowing in nursing. *Advances in Nursing Science*, *1*(1), 13-23.

Chinn, P. L., & Jacobs, M. K. (1987). *Theory and nursing: A systematic approach* (2nd ed.) (Chapters 1 and 2, pp. 1-62). St. Louis: Mosby.

Silva, M. C. & Rothbart, D. (1984, January). An analysis of changing trends in philosophies of science on nursing theory development and testing. *Advances in Nursing Science*, *6*(2), 1-13. (See also Letter to the Editor in *ANS 9*(2), January 1987.)

Learning Activities:

Continue work on personal journal.

Begin exploring topics for scholarly essay.

Suggestion: Make a list of "burning questions" about nursing and your specialty area of practice, and begin discussing them with your colleagues.

WEEK #4

WHAT IS THEORY AND WHY DOES IT EXIST? (OCTOBER 3)

(Course objectives 1.1, 2.1)

Conveners:_____

Readings:

Bunch, C. (1987). Not by degrees: Feminist theory and education. In C. Bunch (Ed.), *Passionate politics: Feminist theory in action* (pp. 240-253). New York: St. Martin's Press.

Chinn, P. L., & Jacobs, M. K. (1987). *Theory and nursing: A systematic approach* (2nd ed.) (Chapter 3, pp. 64-85). St. Louis: Mosby.

Kindilien, C. (1982). *Basic writing skills* (Part Four: A Writing Procedure, pp. 71-97). New York: Arco.

Meleis, A. I. (1985). *Theoretical nursing: Development and progress* (Chapter 5, pp. 79-106). Philadelphia: Lippincott.

Stember, M. (1986). Model building as a strategy for theory development. In P. L. Chinn (Ed.), *Nursing research methodology: Issues and implementation* (pp. 103-119). Rockville, MD: Aspen Publishers.

Learning Activities:

Continue work on personal journal.

Work on Stage 1 from Kindilien.

Suggestion: Select one of your "burning questions" and try to frame a main sentence around this question.

WEEK #7

EVALUATION OF THEORY (OCTOBER 24)

(Course Objectives 1.1, 1.6, 4.1, 4.2, 4.3, 4.4)

Conveners:_____

Readings:

Chinn, P. L. & Jacobs, M. K. (1987). *Theory and nursing: A systematic approach* (2nd ed.) (Chapter 6, pp. 134-148). St. Louis: Mosby.

Ramos, M.C. (1987). Adopting an evolutionary lens: An optimistic approach to discovering strength in nursing. *Advances in Nursing Science, 10*(1), 19-26.

Learning Activities:

Continue work on personal journal.

Complete Kindilien's Stage 3.

Suggestion: Kindilien's suggestions are wonderful! Set aside about 3 hours to sit down and do it. Work with a word processor if possible; write no more than about 4 to 5 pages at this stage.

Read what you have written to get a general idea of immediate impressions you want to tend to now, but then let it rest and don't work with it any more.

SHARE DRAFT OF YOUR SCHOLARLY WRITING at the October 24 gathering. Be sure to bring two copies of your work; one for faculty and one for another participant.

WEEK #8

THEORY, PRACTICE, AND RESEARCH LINKS (OCTOBER 31)

(Course objectives 1.4, 1.5, 1.6, 2.1, 3.1, 3.2, 4)

Conveners:_____

Readings:

Benner, P., & Tanner, C. (1987, January). How expert nurses use intuition. *American Journal of Nursing, 87*(1), 23-31.

Chinn, P. L. & Jacobs, M. K. (1987). *Theory and nursing: A systematic approach* (2nd ed.) (Chapters 7 & 8, pp. 150-180). St. Louis: Mosby.

Fawcett, J. (1979, October). The relationship between theory and research: A double-helix. *Advances in Nursing Science, 1*(1), 49-62.

Quinn, J. F. (1984, January). Thrapeutic touch as energy exchange. *Advances in Nursing Science, 6*(2), 42-49.

Learning Activities:

Continue work on personal journal. Complete your critique of your colleague's scholarly writing. Use the adapted ANS review form.

Suggestion: Be constructive. Point out things about the writing that need improvement and offer suggestions for making the changes needed. Don't worry about whether you are "correct" – simply share your impressions with the author. Remember that this is not meant to be a finished product; your comments will help the author to refine the writing. Comment on both the content of the writing and the presentation or style.

SHARE YOUR REVIEW WITH THE AUTHOR AND RETURN THE DRAFT TO THE AUTHOR at the October 31 gathering.

References

Daly, M., & Caputi, J. (1987). *Websters first new intergalactic wickedary of the English language*. Boston: Beacon Press.

Harding, S. (1987). *Feminism and methodology: Social science issues*. Bloomington: Indiana University Press.

Spender, D. (1982). *Invisible women: The schooling scandal*. London: Writers and Readers Publishing Cooperative.

Weiler, K. (1988). *Women teaching for change: Gender, class & power*. South Hadley, MA: Bergin & Garvey.

Wheeler, C. E., & Chinn, P. L. (1984). *Peace and power: A handbook of feminist process*. Buffalo, NY: Margaretdaughters.

Wheeler, C. E., & Chinn, P. L. (1989). Peace *and power: A handbook of feminist process* (2nd ed.). New York: National League for Nursing.

Reflections on Feminist Pedagogy in Nursing Education

Peggy L. Chinn

Things that have changed as well as things that have not changed since I originally wrote this chapter on feminist pedagogy are stunning! From a feminist point of view, we have come a long way, but not nearly far enough. Two significant things that have not changed are related to the intransigence of patriarchal ideologies. Institutions of higher education, like all other major social institutions, remain essentially patriarchal. Deeply embedded patriarchal and hierarchical hegemonies remain entrenched in the consciousness of both teachers and students.

At the same time, feminist perspectives have grown and matured, are widely accepted, and have continued to affect ideologic, social, and political change. The World Wide Web was created, and, once established, skyrocketed to transform communication, access and use of information, and methods of teaching and learning. The definition and practices that constitute literacy have been dramatically transformed from a written word, paper-bound kind of literacy to a literacy that depends on rapid comprehension of electronic images, sounds, and symbols. Yet the world of the Web, and of technology in general, remains primarily a patriarchal domain.

I believe that feminist pedagogy of today and of the future depends upon the maturity of feminist perspectives, combined with creative, feminist-oriented uses of the electronic resources that are now at our fingertips. Taking this path is a powerful choice – a tool that brings about personal and social change. The fundamental philosophy that is explained in the original chapter has matured over the years, as have the teaching methods that have been developed and applied by myself and others. The sections that follow relate what I have learned and practiced in using feminist pedagogy and technology since the original chapter was published.

Evidence Supporting Feminist Pedagogy

A number of colleagues who were once enrolled in doctoral courses that I taught began using feminist pedagogies and methods drawn from their experiences working with me. Some of them decided to rise to the challenge of those who pointed to the lack of evidence that supported the claim that feminist pedagogies empowered students or led to personal and social change. Adeline Falk-Rafael led an initiative to conduct a major study, and to publish articles that related experiential and research results related to outcomes of feminist pedagogy (Chinn, 2007; Falk-Rafael, Anderson, Chinn, & Rubotzky, 2004; Falk-Rafael, Chinn, Anderson, Laschinger, & Rubotzky, 2004).

The research study was conducted in classrooms other than my own, in three different colleges and universities, and in prelicensure and master's courses. The particular teaching methods the teachers used drew on *Peace and Power* (Chinn, 2007) and were consistent with the "powers" described in the original chapter in this book. However, each of the teachers in the courses involved in the research study adapted these approaches according to the circumstances of their particular curriculum and setting. *Peace and Power* is not prescriptive; rather it presents a feminist and value-based perspective that guides the creation of particular teaching methods. This is a significant aspect of the research led by Falk-Rafael. Despite the variability in the three diverse settings, and the variability of teachers, the results of the research are compelling. The findings of the study supported two hypotheses: that empowerment would increase over the course of the class in which feminist pedagogy was used, and that classroom empowerment extended beyond the classroom to personal and work situations (Falk-Rafael et al., 2003).

The Difficult Challenge: Grading and Feminist Pedagogy

An even more urgent challenge than that of evidence concerning outcomes of feminist pedagogy has been the very real challenge that grading and grading practices are inherently patriarchal, and that this process sets up a difficult power-over relationship between teachers and students. Teachers who use feminist pedagogy generally have no doubt that our approaches lead to excellent learning experiences, and we generally have ample (although not universal!) student feedback on course evaluations that support our belief. But I have yet to encounter a teacher who uses feminist pedagogy who is satisfied with the process of grading.

The original article on feminist pedagogy illustrates my early attempts to address the challenge of grading, but it took years for me to begin to resolve many of the underlying issues and reach a certain level of peace with this process. I began to seriously tackle the issue of articulating a feminist praxis for grading once I found Nel Noddings' philosophy of education, and read her wonderful book *Women and Evil* (Noddings, 1989, 1995). It was very exciting to find philosophic support for bringing together a fundamental nursing value – caring – with feminist pedagogy!

Noddings' philosophic views and explanations of what caring is and how it is expressed ethically in human relationships provided the foundation for developing a philosophy of nursing education (Chinn, 1999), and a praxis for grading (Chinn, 2004). These works retain the focus on the "powers" of *Peace and Power* as the foundation for a grading praxis – the synergistic reflection and action to transform what has been to grading practices that flow from the "peace powers."

The practices that I describe (one from a freshman course "Introduction to Health", and another from a doctoral course) are only examples; the approach is not prescriptive. There are many other possibilities for specific approaches to grading, and the approaches vary with the educational objectives and learning level of the students (Chinn, 2004). Regardless of the specific approach to grading, the changes that occur in the practices of grading shift the focus from getting assignments (often busywork) completed for a grade to understanding the underlying value and reason for engaging in various learning activities. The practices "call forth the best" in every student (consistent with Noddings' philosophy), rather than police or oversee what might be "wrong." Feminist grading practices open the way for students to fully exercise their own powers of responsibility, creativity, nurturing, and diversity (in their own individuality). Faculty fulfill their responsibility to model their best nursing practices, to guide students in achieving the knowledge and skills required to be a well-prepared nurse, and to share specific feedback and assistance with each student achievement.

The World Wide Web and Distance Learning

The World Wide Web, which literally did not exist when I wrote the original chapter, has dramatically changed the entire world, including teaching and learning. At that time, the Internet had begun to develop and we were beginning to use a very awkward form of email, but few envisioned the possibilities created by the World Wide Web. Tim Berners-Lee, who created the underlying structure from which the web is built, had and still has a well-articulated set of values from which his vision of the web grew. He was committed to democratic values that assure equal, universal, worldwide access to a wealth of information, that nurture diversity, sound social interactions, and empowerment for all. In his book that describes the design of the web and his vision for its future, he says:

> The web is more a social creation than a technical one. I designed it for a social effect to help people work together and not as a technical toy. The ultimate goal of the web is to support and improve our web like existence in the world. We clump together into families, associations, and companies. We develop trust across the miles and distrust around the corner. What we believe, endorse, agree with, and depend on is representable and, increasingly, represented on the Web. We all have to ensure that the society we build with the Web is of the sort we intend (Berners-Lee, 2000, p. 123).

Teaching approaches online that use feminist pedagogies contribute precisely to this … building the sort of social communities in nursing that we intend.

I began my earliest trials with distance learning simply using email, combined with face-to-face classroom meetings. The first course that I taught only online was an elective doctoral course on "Feminism and Nursing". At the time that I taught that course in the spring of 1996, the World Wide Web had just begun to emerge on a broad scale. Windows 95 had just been released the previous August, and browsers to access the Web had not yet been routinely installed or packaged as standard software on new computers.

The course did have a rudimentary Web page, and my intention at the outset was to use the website to post information such as the class roster with email addresses, shared readings, the syllabus, and other course materials. I had also intended for students to share their drafts of scholarly writing on the web. As it turned out, while all of the students did have access to the web, it was difficult to use and even more difficult for me to maintain the site (there were no web design WYSIWYG programs!). Given the small size of the class (6 students), we ended up using email for class discussions, and getting materials to everyone on paper using snail mail, since email could not yet easily transfer attachments to everyone.

We used *Peace and Power* processes as the structure for our email discussions. Every week everyone sent a message to the group that included their check-in for the week. The convener for the week (a participant each week on a rotating basis) posted a SOPHIA. SOPHIA is an acronym for Speak Out, Play Havoc, Imagine Alternatives. It is a brief personal essay (not a summary of the readings) that challenges everyone in the class to think critically about the readings and about the issues we are discussing, and ends with "subjectives" – questions that help stimulate and focus the discussion. Everyone entered into the discussion stimulated by the SOPHIA and the shared readings for the week. At the end of the week, everyone sent a closing message.

Since that first experience, I have taught many courses using the World Wide Web, email, online discussion boards, and telecom connections for distance synchronous classes. In all instances, I have been able to use similar *Peace and Power* structures for discussions and class interactions. As an example, I taught a first-year course "Introduction to Health" required for all nursing majors, and open to any other student in the University. It was offered simultaneously on four different campuses throughout the state of Connecticut. We used the simultaneous meetings to introduce new concepts related to health, then shifted to online discussions during the week. Small groups worked on projects using email and WebCT groups. We adapted check-in and closing so that students on local campuses interacted to get acquainted with one another, and provided closing messages online regularly throughout the semester. Since discussion that includes every participant is very difficult in synchronous distance situations, using principles of having every voice heard was valuable to reinforce to everyone that even on a television screen, their opinion and ideas count!

My preference is a combination of online and face-to-face classrooms; I have not found synchronous teaching and learning to be effective or beneficial, and not worth the expense and investment required of the institution. If I had to make a choice between online and face-to-face contexts for any one class, I would choose the online classroom because of several major advantages it has provided in putting into action many of the ideals of feminist pedagogy. I do stress that my preference remains a combination, because of the personal connection that only face-to-face interactions can provide. But the advantages of online teaching and learning are many for enacting feminist pedagogies, and for building the kinds of scholarly communities in nursing that we intend.

One of the most obvious advantages of online learning is that every individual has equal access to "speaking" without interruption, limited only by individual skill, patience, and courage to "e-speak." In my experience, this feature has provided, over and over again, a voice for students who are silenced in the face-to-face classroom. For example, on many occasions, students who represent a minority (sometimes an invisible minority in face-to-face classrooms) have spoken their own "truth" online in ways they would never dare to speak face-to-face. In the first two courses I taught using online discussion, minority students shared a point of view about the readings that were at great odds with that of the majority of the students. In both instances, the majority of the students were taken aback by the minority viewpoint – some did not understand it, or tried to discount it or "correct" the minority student.

I learned from those two early encounters that one of the teaching skills that I needed to develop was online mediation that provided support to the minority student, helping to bridge understandings in ways that affirmed rather than discounted any person's perceived reality, but also nurturing new insight and understanding. I also learned to lay the foundation even stronger at the outset of any course concerning the intention of our discussions – the values of honoring diversity, of treating one another with respect, and being committed to fully understanding views with which we do not agree. I ultimately came to see this as a balance between creating safety and freedom as co-existing conditions for excellence in online teaching (Chinn, 2003).

Another advantage of online teaching is the "space" it provides for solitude that nurtures depth. At the same time, online learning provides reliable transfer and sharing of everyone's thoughts and ideas, which in turn nurtures a broad range of feedback that "corrects" or affirms the ideas. This is particularly important for graduate education, where we seek to nurture a depth and breadth of knowledge, and ultimately the student's ability to contribute unique, well-developed ideas to a broad audience. Online learning, in a context of feminist pedagogy,

- encourages each student to develop their own ideas and thinking (which requires solitude and personal investment of study, thought, and creativity),
- supports each student in sharing their ideas in early draft forms as well as in closer-to-completion forms, and
- nurtures each student's ability to become a skilled critic of one another's ideas and scholarship.

Another advantage of online learning is that it provides the opportunity to broaden the "classroom" to the student's own community. In the absence of face-to-face connections with others who are enrolled in the course, I have often designed learning activities that take each student to their own community. They are prompted to discuss issues related to the course, gather experiential information, explore areas of their community that might have been invisible to them before this course, and/or compare what they are learning in readings and discussions with what they observe in their communities. As each student engages with their community, they bring their observations and insights to the course discussion, which enriches the learning for everyone in the class. Of course, these same kinds of learning activities can be part of a face-to-face course as well, but I have found that these activities take on a new meaning for students in an online course. The connection with the "real world" takes on a special meaning that contrasts sharply with the virtual reality of the class, and the activity is far less likely to seem like busywork; instead, it becomes the necessary link between the lofty world of ideas and the swampy world of practice.

The last issue I will address is one major challenge in teaching online – it can and often does take an immense investment of teacher time and energy, especially when it is designed using feminist pedagogy. Every voice being heard, for example, without time constraints, could fill a thousand-page novel! So I learned very early to find ways to protect my own time and energy; to place clear limits on expectations of time and energy that each participant, including myself as teacher, would invest; to structure ways that demystified my own role and responsibilities. For example, I designate one day a week that I will not be available online and ask everyone else to also designate a day off for themselves (the power of nurturing). I typically only respond to the group, not to individual discussion postings (the power of the whole). I set up clear guidelines and timelines, all of which can be renegotiated with the group, but that give us all a starting point for what we expect of one another (the power of responsibility).

Where to from Here?

Over the years, I have grown in my understanding of what it means to be a feminist teacher, to translate what this means in ways that students of all different persuasions can understand and reach an appreciation of an experience crafted with feminist values at the center. It has been a deeply satisfying journey. It also continues to offer immense challenges, and there are the same kinds of difficulties that come with any approach to teaching and learning. The process of addressing the challenges and difficulties with a firm foundation of feminist values is a teacher's own "classroom" – an ongoing, life-long learning that draws on the growing feminist literature resources, maturing theoretical and philosophic nursing perspectives, and the experience of doing it.

In my view, nursing education needs feminist pedagogies now more than ever before – pedagogies that value diversity, promote more inclusive sharing and interaction, and model cooperative (not competitive) ways of working together. We need more research evidence that enacting these values in the classroom has the effects we seek. We need a host of new ideas for teaching methods that are grounded in feminist and nursing values. If nurse educators do anything to contribute to the health and well-being of individuals and societies, we must do it in our classrooms. Feminist pedagogies are consistent with nursing values. Using these approaches, we teach and model ways of communicating, interacting, and working together that nurture each person's highest potential, high-level wellness, and harmony within their communities.

References

Berners-Lee, T. (2000). *Weaving the Web: The original design and the ultimate destiny of the World Wide Web*. New York: Harper Business.

Chinn, P. L. (1999). A Philosophy of Nursing Education. [Slide show.] Retrieved from http://ans-info.net/Caring%20curriculum_files/frame.htm

Chinn, P. L. (2003). Teaching creativity online. *Annual Review of Nursing Education, 1*, 199-207.

Chinn, P. L. (2004). A praxis for grading. In M. H. Oermann & K. T. Heinrich (Eds.), *Annual review of nursing education, Vol. 2* (pp. 89-109). New York: Springer Publishing.

Chinn, P. L. (2007). *Peace and power: Creative leadership for building communities* (6th ed.). Boston: Jones & Bartlett.

Falk-Rafael, A. R., Anderson, M. A., Chinn, P. L., & Rubotzky, A. M. (2004). Peace and power as a critical feminist framework for nursing education. In M. H. Oermann & K. T. Heinrich (Eds.), *Annual review of nursing education, Vol. 2* (pp. 217-235). New York: Springer Publishing.

Falk-Rafael, A. R., Chinn, P. L., Anderson, M. A., Laschinger, H., & Rubotzky, A. M. (2004). The effectiveness of feminist pedagogy in empowering a community of learners. *Journal of Nursing Education, 43*(3), 107-115.

Noddings, N. (1989). *Women and evil*. Berkeley, CA: University of California Press.

Noddings, N. (1995). *Philosophy of education*. Boulder, CO: Westview Press.

Reflecting on Revolutions: A Half-Century in Nursing Education

Verle Waters

Reflecting is something people in my age group do a lot. One of the aims of the age-appropriate occupation of reflecting on the past is to tease out the persistent threads that bring coherence to all the decades now past that were inevitably filled with twists and turns and ups and downs. Finding underlying coherence is satisfying – discovering that the journey from then to now wasn't as piecemeal and random as it seemed at times, brings both comfort and a new understanding. Is there underlying coherence in the journey nursing education has taken in the past half-century? And within the somersaults of my own career in that arena? I decide that there is progression in the former and consistency in the latter: broadly speaking there were revolutionary changes in nursing education, and I had my turns at the barricades.

I began my study of nursing during World War II, and became a teacher in 1952. 1952 was a time of yawning shortage in nursing, and the remedy initiated by nursing leaders was a revolutionary change in the educational program in order to increase the supply of nurses. Seven pilot programs to educate nurses in the community junior college changed nursing forever. I was lucky enough to be the first full-time teacher in the initial program at Orange County Community College in Middletown, New York. That experience shaped my mind-set about education and prefigured the career that lay ahead. We, the teachers in the pilot programs, had all the attributes of a cell group: we were overthrowing entrenched beliefs, practices, and regulations. It was thrilling work. In a complete overhaul, the new programs changed location of the educational program, the structure of learning activities, and the population of nursing students. Now, looking back, I can see that location, structure, and population are recurring issues in discussions of programs preparing nurses, and the calls for change in the decades since often revolve around these same topics.

Shortage and surplus periodically recur in nursing, and nursing education is called upon to remedy both. We are, as everyone knows, now challenged again by a shortage of such dimensions that it is a topic in the national media. Within recent weeks even I have had a phone call from a nurse recruiter, and a glitzy invitation from the U.S. Army offering me the opportunity to realize a new future. Education is again under pressure to respond (a better bet than phone calls to people like me). In 1952, the remedy was to create a sustainable, supportable program that would accept and appeal to a new population of students. The relatively small number of baccalaureate programs and an even smaller number of graduate programs at that time could not have satisfied the need. The picture is dramatically different now.

Twenty years later – by now there were over 600 ADN programs – there was a nursing surplus, and new graduates now hunted and waited for job openings. Just as my career identity was shaped by my engagement in the radical associate degree program in that time of a dramatic post-war shortage, so, too, during the period of surplus, I chose to mount the barricades when the American Nurses Association conducted a vigorous campaign to end the licensing of ADN graduates as registered nurses. New legislation was being introduced state by state to require the baccalaureate degree for the RN license and channel associate degree and practical nurse programs into a merger. (The cause and effect relationship between nursing surplus or shortage and the pitch of so-called Entry into Practice activity is one that I make; others may see it differently.) In February 1978, I was invited to present a paper at an ANA conference entitled "Entry into Practice" and held in Kansas City. It was the most anxiety-inducing invitation I ever had; I accepted, and obsessed over my preparation. I had been a member of the committee that created the 1965 ANA Position Paper that called for two levels of nursing practice: professional and technical. Each was expressly linked to the two college-based programs. My assigned topic was "Progress of the Nursing Profession in Implementing the Position Paper" and my intention was to support, still, the concept of differential roles but disagree with a method that disfranchised ADN graduates. I had learned by then that I am not good at confrontation. Aggressive language ties up my own tongue. But I am a persuader, with great admiration for the power of words. I went to Kansas City to persuade. There was a terrible snowstorm that almost paralyzed Kansas City and surrounding states. I had been skiing with a son in Utah, and the flight to Kansas City on a small propeller plane through blinding snow was among the most nerve-jangling rides of my life. And then, for reasons related to the storm that I can't remember, I could not properly show a set of graphs I had laboriously prepared. Still, re-reading that paper now, I secretly think it is quite good.

I try now to remember the motivation that drove me into that literal and metaphoric snowstorm. Of course, I clearly thought that I was right. As much as I agreed, from the beginning, that differential work roles for graduates of the two programs was important and desirable, the ANA-proposed solution was unthinkable. I argued in Kansas City that nursing service held the key to differential work roles, and got a little carried away by my own words in making the argument. I said

> *The unique professional nursing role, as sketched in the position paper and elaborated in the years since, has for many educators substance, promise, and conviction; however, the role dims as it moves out of the language of education into the language of nursing service. It continues to lose precision as it moves from community settings in through the doors of the acute hospital. It begins to vaporize as it drifts from the teaching hospital in urban centers out through the suburbs until, on reaching the 75 bed hospital in a small town, it is a diffuse and foreign notion.*

What bothered me the most, and prompted me to elbow my way to the barricades again in the 1980s when I became aware of the Curriculum Revolution, was the degree of estrangement between AD educators and higher degree faculty brought about by the Entry into Practice wars and the negative effects of estrangement. It had not always been that way. In California in the early 1960s, new programs were developing in both community colleges and four-year colleges, and there were both formal and informal get-togethers of faculty from both programs making an agreeable (if not terribly conclusive) effort to understand what was the same and what was different in the set of nursing courses in each program.

In those many discussions to clarify in good faith the proper playing field for each of our programs, the deliberations were earnest, and focused, always, on "content." This is your content," we said to each other, and "this is ours." Agreement was difficult, and precision elusive. It was an all-day session in San Francisco and the comment by Marian McDermott, a teacher in the San Francisco City College ADN program that made me first think about the red-herring role that "content" played in the search for differences between the two programs, and handicapped our efforts to make changes in our own programs. I can't remember the sponsorship of this particular all-day session; it was, I believe, held at UCSF. There was a room full of participants, 15 or 20 teachers from each type of program. Marlene Kramer presided and began the day presenting a case – a child with third-degree burns over most of his body. She described his condition in detail, including laboratory, observational, and cultural data, and then sent us in work-alike groups to outline the content that would be taught in our particular program regarding the care of this little boy. We came back with pages of content thought to be essential in preparing our particular graduate, and group after group reported as Marlene filled sheets of Flipchart paper with notes. When reports were finished, we pondered the results, hoping for enlightenment as we compared "their" list with "ours." Marion raised her hand, stood (she is majestically tall) and said, "I've concluded that the major difference between associate and baccalaureate degree programs is the vocabulary of the faculty." We laughed, but her observation was an epiphany for me. Content is not the answer.

In 1972, Sonoma State College in California opened what I believe to be among the first baccalaureate programs designed specifically and exclusively for students who were RNs. In the 1960s and 1970s, programs offering a baccalaureate degree to RNs were a hodge-podge, of very uneven quality. Some required RNs to take the full four-year generic program, others offering no nursing courses at all, but awarded a bachelor's degree after two years of lower division general education. Mary Searight at Sonoma State developed an upper division two-year course of study that assumed a basis of lower division nursing study. I worked with her and her faculty as curriculum consultant to offer a basis for answering the critical question: what is upper division nursing that is not lower division nursing? In a chapter I contributed to Mary Searight's book on her project, I noted the "concerned ambivalence" nursing educators have toward change. I observed that "the sense that educational programs have been artificially rigid and unresponsive to students as individuals co-exists with a fear that to make the programs otherwise will lower standards, dilute quality, and devalue nursing and nursing care."

As the Entry into Practice conflict heated up, associate degree educators responded by withdrawing from participation in the national organizations, forming a new organization for ADN educators, and seeing adversaries where once they had seen friends. In addition, I believe faculty responded by battening down the hatches, so to speak, making the curriculum less experimental, more traditional, and more fully packed with blessed content. It was a self-protective response.

Then I began listening to the Curriculum Revolutionaries. It was a pick-up group that started with Em Bevis, Nancy Diekelmann, Chris Tanner, and others. They were talking about reforming nursing education. They were all associated with baccalaureate and graduate programs, but their rallying cries were as important to associate degree faculty as any, and I wanted to join them on the barricades.

The NLN was admirably responsive, publishing a series of small booklets on the topic, producing at least one videotape, enrolling speakers on the topic at meetings, and sponsoring at least one get-together of the revolutionaries. The revolutionary mantra was an assault on rigid classroom protocols, lectures, and "covering content." I listened to and participated in the discussions about enlarging the sense of community, incorporating new pedagogies, changing the relationship between teacher and student, and responding to a changing student population. There is an echo of the goals set forth in the 1952 educational revolution: a fruitful location of the learning enterprise, an effective structure of learning activities, and sensitivity to a diverse student population. But the shape of the challenges was new, more complex, and better understood.

I try, in reflecting on revolutions I have known, to pin down the long-term effect on me of participating in that heady period of conferences and conversations. I have a copy of a videotape made by NLN on which David Allen, Em Bevis, Peggy Chinn and I, inspirited by Pat Moccia, exchange words on the topic "Curriculum Revolutions and Counterrevolutions." First, I look longingly at how I looked 20 years ago, compared to the face I see in the mirror today. Then I wonder whatever happened to that suit, which I barely remember. Finally, listening to the words, I consider the evolution of my own beliefs and actions in the nearly 25 years I spent as a program director and curriculum consultant.

Along the way I gained new insights of use in my work. There are maxims about faculty-student relationships in the Curriculum Revolution that are equally applicable to director-teacher relationships. On the videotape, Em Bevis is eloquent about the uses of power in the academic enterprise and she argues for power-sharing between teacher and student, an argument as suited to the director-teacher duo. Early in my practice in an education leadership role, I recognized that you do not set out to change the person and indeed you cannot, but the leader can change circumstances and situations, and foster change in the teacher's actions as a result. Finding time and settings for faculty to come together is a challenge, sometimes requiring the leader to beg, borrow, or steal to obtain a day or days and a place where the easy flow of ideas and words occurs. Most faculty members already have all the good ideas tucked away somewhere, but they don't come out because Who Knows? they might not be well-received. Once expressed and examined, the best become realized. But for them to even be expressed, there has to be freedom to voice all of the ideas, the bad ones, the pet peeves, and the favorite hobby horses. It has been my experience that the good ideas will rise like cream rises on unpasteurized milk.

Early in the 1980s, before anyone we knew was doing it, the Ohlone College faculty discussed enlisting selected staff nurses as preceptors for senior students. An exploratory meeting with staff nurses and the director of nursing moved the idea along. As we sat working with the wonderful staff nurses who would become preceptors, mentors, and role models for our students, I reflected on the change in the education-service relationship going on around me. Thirty-five years earlier, nursing education declared itself divorced from nursing service; now here we were making nice and wanting reconciliation. Both of us had grown up in those 35 years, and I knew this marriage was going to work. The preceptorship was and is a great success, helped immeasurably in inception by a grant from W.K. Kellogg, which provided time and means for planning, coaching, developing structure and written materials, and putting an evaluation protocol in place.

Around the same time, another Aha! moment came my way that led to an at least quasi-revolutionary project. I was in a small group session here in California, listening to a young teacher explain how she had structured her adult med-surg course around a carefully chosen set of case studies. I admired what she was doing and it sounded as if she was engaging her students in appealing and effective learning experiences built around the cases. But the oldest prototypical patient in her set was a 50-year-old man who had had a heart attack. Even though I was perfectly healthy, I was (and am) female and over 50, and I wanted her students to know something about me if I did end up in their care. I didn't actually think that, but the sense of what is missing if you stop thinking about nursing needs before you get to the old chronically ill population was jarring. I knew we were doing better at Ohlone, but our focus, too, was on the hospitalized patient. We had a few faculty conversations where the realists pointed out the challenges in finding and structuring clinical experiences with patients in nursing homes and the community. Challenges included the quality of nursing home care, commonly held attitudes toward the patients therein, staffing levels, and more. No one denied that, given population and health care trends, students needed more gerontology and perhaps more experience with the long-term care population. We knew that extended care facilities had been and were sometimes used for brief skill-building student experiences early in the program of study, and we reasoned that a late-program experience would bring students to those settings with greater sensibility and skill, and, equally important, probably have an impact on the skill level of the staff in the agency. This was clearly bigger than a one-school project.

I went to an NLN meeting while those thoughts were buzzing in my head, and ran into Susan Sherman from the Community College of Philadelphia sitting in the hotel lobby. I brought up to her the idea of something along the lines of a two-coast project to promote gerontology and the nursing home in associate degree programs. It was the first of many conversations that led in time to a seven-year project supported by funds from the W.K. Kellogg Foundation. The Robert Wood Johnson-funded Teaching Nursing Home project had enabled baccalaureate and graduate schools of nursing to establish clinical teaching affiliations with large nursing homes; we felt there was a place for a somewhat parallel project to enable affiliations between associate degree nursing programs (there were 780 at the time) and small community nursing homes. Six colleges, representing both coasts, the Middle West, and the Rocky Mountain region became demonstration sites, The six demonstration sites mounted outreach activities in their region. The design of the Community College-Nursing Home Partnership, as the project was called, was inspired by a Ford Foundation project that I had read about many years earlier and never forgot. Intended to improve public school education, the Ford project initiated major changes in a few schools selected because they were strong, were seen to be influential and were spread across the country. Ford called them Lighthouse Schools: the title alone conveys their role.

The years of working with the faculty in my own school and five others in that period yielded a few more insights – call them principles – about being an effective faculty leader when moving toward the positive side of that "concerned ambivalence" teeter-totter. Curriculum change starts with faculty development, not with the curriculum, and the entire faculty needs to participate in planning development activities. It's important to know who the informal leader is (or leaders are): that is, who the members of the faculty really listen to. If informal leaders do not go along with the plan, it's dead. I found it important to acknowledge the pressure and responsibility a nursing program and its faculty have, and to remember that identity as a nurse is tightly tied to the knowledge base of practice, which, in our curricula, we shovel around from place to place. That's content.

Nursing education studies itself intensely and constantly, and opinions about what should happen next are often exhortations, sometimes leading to revolution. The changes in my lifetime have been stunning, and I wish there was time in the educational programs of today to learn more about that past. I enjoy talking about the yesterdays. When the faculty reluctantly allocated a little class time to me, I sometimes told students about the ritual in my student days for preparing an injection of morphine. They listened, and indulged me, but since that was never going to be on the test, I don't think they cared much about give over have, the glass syringe, the alcohol lamp, and the morphine in tablet form. There is a tendency in me and my age mates to tell the old stories too many times. Nonetheless, it has been an interesting exercise for me to reflect on my past within nursing education and what it has taught me. I have one last piece of advice: never turn your back on a revolution.

On Revolutions and Revolutionaries:
25 Years of Reform and Innovation in Nursing Education
Looking to the Future

M. Elaine Tagliareni and Beverly Malone

the one thing that matters is whether
...the dialogue...before us, be it written
or spoken or neither, remains constantly coming.
(Heidegger, 1971, p. 52)

Leaders of the Curriculum Revolution, whose words echo throughout this book, invited nurse educators, more than two decades ago, to begin a dialogue that was risky and unconventional. They asked nurse educators to talk about change and to legitimatize the understanding that reform was needed in nursing education. Their words and writings stimulated cutting edge thinking about how teachers teach and how students learn. They asked the nursing education community to be open to new ideas and to embrace the teaching of inquiry, reflection, criticism, creativity, and caring. They were considered to be radical thinkers and thoughtful advocates of reform, but dramatic change and transformation, at the instructional and curricular levels of nursing education, never fully materialized. As is true in all revolutions, they were celebrated by some and marginalized by most.

But existing on the margins offers the possibility to see the center differently, to imagine creative alternatives, to resist traditional viewpoints. By being on the margins, these revolutionaries saw the world of nursing education with a new lens. They changed the dialogue about teaching and learning and curriculum development. They urged us to keep the dialogue focused on the current practice environment and on new research, no matter how controversial and uncertain. We are indebted to them for their resilience, for their thoughtful advocacy of nursing's moral commitment to society's need for a competent and efficient nursing workforce, and for their steadfastness to bring excellence to nursing education.

The NLN is proud of the role we played to support and advance the curriculum revolution. As the national nursing organization dedicated to promoting excellence at every level of nursing education, the NLN continues to advocate for the voices of nurse educators who seek to move from the margins to the center and who are critical catalysts, attuned to the best of what the center has to offer while clearly aligning themselves with colleagues who are dedicated to keep alive potent traditions of critique and dialogue (West, 1990). As with any revolution, the origins of the Curriculum Revolution were shaped and formed in the reservoir of tradition existing within and alongside the needs and demands of a changing world. In the spirit of the Curriculum Revolutionaries, who paved the way for consideration of grassroots efforts to enlighten and foster strategic change, it is the NLN's goal to promote continued dialogue about curriculum reform, recognizing that questioning and sustained critique lead to new understandings between individuals, groups, communities, and, particularly for nursing, between the practice of nursing and the education of the practitioners.

The Impetus for Reform

The work of these revolutionaries was far-reaching and zealous. Bevis (see Chapter 3) and Diekelmann (see Chapter 1) challenged the time-honored Tyler model, which placed high value on certainty and predictability, as well as on accumulation of facts, principles, classifications, and theories that can be explained deductively. This was the gold standard at the time. Diekelmann pointed out that the traditional model of nursing education de-emphasized the "here and now" and that crowded, content-laden curricula hindered opportunities for dialogue with students by providing little beyond the provision or simple transmission of information. She challenged faculty to reframe the belief that educators have "failed" when the curriculum is modified every semester, pointing out that keeping the curriculum current and flexible promotes openness, possibility, and a connection to the reality of the here and now. Even more dramatically, both Bevis and Diekelmann suggested that classroom and clinical courses do not need to have a corresponding relationship, since developing clinical expertise depends on practice and intuitive knowing.

Extending this dialogue, Tanner (see Chapter 5) presented the radical possibility that the technical model of higher education for the professions may not be the most functional in terms of preparing skilled clinicians. She suggested that it was time to examine untested assumptions that practice is only rigorous problem solving accomplished through the application of scientific principles and that the only important and "true" knowledge for practice is derived from research. These were radical ideas for nurses and nurse educators, who listened and recognized, from the center, that aspects of the reform movement were needed. Nonetheless, the belief in traditional models was too powerful, and the call to reform failed to mobilize large groups of nurse educators to achieve transformational change at the national level.

It is not, we believe, that nurse educators failed to recognize that nursing curricula must be well aligned with changes arising from health care reorganization. The overriding purpose of nursing education is and has always been to prepare individuals to meet the health care needs of the public. Certainly, this is an intrinsic value that has consistently characterized reform in nursing education. From its earliest days, the NLN has been at the forefront of these reform efforts to transform nursing education (see the Introduction). Most recently, the NLN's position paper on *Innovation in Nursing Education: A Call to Reform* (2003) called for nursing faculty to revise traditional definitions of innovation away from a long-held belief that innovation is synonymous with the addition of new content, and to embrace innovative practices that speak to developing and using alternative pedagogies. In 2005, the NLN developed a second position paper, *Transforming Nursing Education,* and called for new models of nursing education to emerge, recognizing that we can no longer rely on tradition, past practices, and good intentions. The NLN recommended that proposed changes to nursing programs should emanate from evidence that substantiates the science of nursing education, that provides the foundation for best educational practices, and that meets the needs of the public. A third position paper, *Mentoring of Nurse Faculty* (NLN, 2006), focused on the need to guide new faculty, recognizing the complexity of the faculty role and the need to foster teaching, research, and service skills that facilitate development of future leaders in nursing and nursing education. Within this context – that reform in nursing education must involve a commitment to faculty development in an environment where curriculum redesign is more that a rearrangement of content and must be research based – the NLN has consistently understood and valued its mission to build a strong nursing workforce through excellence and innovation, at all levels of nursing education.

Currently, driving forces in the health care environment necessitate renewed energy directed toward significant reform. There is growing awareness that nursing education cannot expect to increase capacity with traditional models. Adding schools or increasing enrollment will not solve the problem, especially in light of the growing faculty shortage, institutional limits within programs, and decreasing number of clinical sites. In addition, there is a renewed appreciation that health care education needs redesign. What is reasonable to expect from nursing education? For instance, is simulation a transformational step in the process of developing improved thinking skills of graduates? With increased errors, high turnover rates of new graduates in acute care, and concern that nursing graduates do not embrace decision making that leads to accountability for the continuation of care, there is wide understanding that different and enhanced competencies are needed by nursing graduates at all levels of education (Del Bueno, 2005; IOM 1996, 2006). Furthermore, there is growing awareness that current articulation models have not motivated or enticed students in entry level programs to pursue advanced study. How will new statewide initiatives (such as those in Oregon, New York, Texas, and Connecticut) change the landscape of curricular design? Will these initiatives foster more affordable and accessible seamless career pathways? Indeed, the contemporary call to reform in nursing education is far reaching.

Bringing Renewed Voice to Nursing Education

Since the heady days of the Curriculum Revolution, faculty across the country have instituted reform on a local level; pockets of innovation have sprung up in schools of nursing as nurse educators have embraced the recommendations of the curriculum revolution, as well as newer ideas about interactive teaching styles and interpretive pedagogies (e.g., Benner,

Tanner, & Chesla, 1996; Diekelmann, 2001; Ironside, 2005, 2006; Tanner, 2002a, 2002b). To encourage these innovative steps, the NLN has created a program designed to identify Centers of Excellence in Nursing Education. As an entire School of Nursing takes up the role of being a Center of Excellence, the marginal revolutionary approaches have the opportunity to become integrated into and identified with a new "center." Certainly more and more nursing faculty are taking up the call to reform and moving it from the margins to the mainstream. While there are many focused hotbeds of creativity and transformation, overall substantive reform of curriculum in nursing education remains on the margins.

How will nurse educators embrace the movement toward renewed reform and find a balance between mainstream, time-honored models and new ideas, while finding energy in new perspectives? In other words, how can we change the bathwater without throwing out the baby? We know that the NLN will continue to support the dynamic tension between center and margin, recognizing our potential to provide a foundation and a forum for critical debate and discussion. This is the essence of the challenge for the NLN, as the professional voice for nurse educators. And it resonates with the mandate established decades ago by the Curriculum Revolutionaries as they boldly envisioned a new way of practicing based on what we as nurses *know*, not on what we *do*.

The NLN's current strategic plan calls for enhancing the NLN's national and international impact as the recognized leader in nursing education and for committing itself to be a diverse, member-led organization that champions nurse educators in political, academic and professional arenas. The advancement of the science of nursing education, through promotion of evidence-based nursing education and the scholarship of teaching, continues to be at the forefront of NLN decision making about future initiatives. As leaders of the NLN, we are committed to making certain that, in every decision we make on behalf of the organization, we are contributing in a meaningful way to building a nursing workforce that is competent, ethical, caring, diverse, and sustainable. At the forefront of this commitment is recognition that to be a truly effective professional voice for our members, we must create mechanisms to invite dialogue that offers new and differing perspectives, to use information from the margins to transform the way we think about the whole (hooks, 1990; Guinier, Fine, & Balin, 1997).

To accomplish this we will look to the past and celebrate its lessons. The NLN and its members will stand on the shoulders of our colleagues who dared to speak from the margins in an effort to bring new perspectives and radical possibility to the center. We have so much to learn from previous attempts at curricular reform; there is a richness of dialogue and ideas that will lay the groundwork for future directions. But to create new models for curriculum development and reform in the future, we understand that we must find new ways to generate positive and enduring change that is the essence of transformation.

As the NLN implements its mission to promote excellence in nursing education to develop a strong and diverse nursing workforce, we are emboldened by the needs of today's health care system to fully understand how individuals experience and respond to health and illness, to explore what individuals and families most value in their daily lives, and which aspects of their lives are most significant to maintaining function and cultural integrity. We fully recognize that fostering quality and safety education in all nursing programs is the pathway to advocacy for those most vulnerable. To reiterate the words of Bevis (see Chapter 3), we will think differently in ways that alter "our perception of teaching and the role of the teacher; that abandons the industrial metaphor; that restructures the relative roles of classroom and clinical practice; that de-emphasizes curriculum development and concentrates on faculty development; that develops a national strategy for change; and, above all, that provides new guideposts for a new age." This message, and others gathered in this volume, resonates today as they did years ago. We will embrace dialogue and critique to give voice to our members as we move the conversations away from the margins to build a new vision for the future of nursing education. For us, this is not a leadership choice, but a leadership imperative.

References

Benner, P. A., Tanner, C. A., & Chesla, C. A. (1996). *Expertise in nursing practice: Caring, clinical judgment, and ethics.* New York: Springer Publishing.

Bevis, E. O. & Watson, J. (1989). *Toward a caring curriculum: A new pedagogy for nursing.* New York: National League for Nursing Press.

Del Bueno, D. (2005). A crisis in critical thinking. *Nursing Education Perspectives, 26*, 278-282.

Diekelmann, N. L. (2001). Narrative pedagogy: Heideggerian hermeneutical analyses of lived experiences of students, teachers, and clinicians. *Advances in Nursing Science, 23*(3), 53-71.

Guinier, L., Fine, M., & Balin, J. (1997). *Becoming gentlemen.* Boston: Beacon Press.

Heidegger, M. (1971). A dialogue on language (P. Hertz, Trans.). In *On the way to language* (pp. 1-54). New York: Harper & Row. (Original work published in 1959)

hooks, b. (1990). Marginality as site of resistance. In R. Ferguson, M. Gever, T. Minh-ha, & C. West (Eds). *Out there: Marginalization and contemporary cultures* (pp. 341-344). Cambridge, MA: MIT Press.

Institute of Medicine. (1996). *Crossing the quality chasm: The IOM health care quality initiative.* http://www.iom.edu/CMS/8089.aspx

Institute of Medicine. (2006). *Preventing medication errors: Quality chasm series.* http://www.iom.edu/CMS/3809/22526/35939.aspx

Ironside, P. M. (2006). Reforming nursing education using Narrative Pedagogy: Learning and practicing interpretive thinking. *Journal of Advanced Nursing, 55,* 478-486.

Ironside, P. M. (2005). Teaching thinking and reaching the limits of memorization: Enacting new pedagogies. *Journal of Nursing Education, 44,* 441-449.

National League for Nursing. (2003). *Innovation in nursing education: A call to reform* (Position statement). New York: Author. http://www.nln.org/aboutnln/PositionStatements/innovation.htm

National League for Nursing. (2005). *Transforming Nursing Education.* (Position Statement). New York: Author. http://www.nln.org/aboutnln/PositionStatements/transforming.htm

National League for Nursing. (2006). *Mentoring of Nurse Faculty.* (Position Statement). New York: Author. http://www.nln.org/aboutnln/PositionStatements/mentoring.htm

Tanner, C. A. (2002a). Clinical education, circa 2010. *Journal of Nursing Education, 41,* 51-52.

Tanner, C. A. (2002b). Education's response to the nursing shortage: Leadership, innovation, and publication. *Journal of Nursing Education, 41,* 467-468.

West, C. (1990). The new cultural politics of difference. In R. Ferguson, M. Gever, T. Minh-ha, & C. West (Eds). *Out there: Marginalization and contemporary cultures* (pp. 19-38). Cambridge, MA: MIT Press.

David G. Allen, PhD, RN, FAAN has focused his work on the intersection of nursing and social justice. In nursing and in women's studies, he teaches methodological issues that arise when power and contested values (especially around systematic disadvantaging by race, class and gender) are central to one's inquiry. Similarly, his theoretical explorations are related to how power, justice, privilege, and disadvantage are embedded in theoretical discourses and what sorts of vocabularies nurses might employ to address these issues directly. Dr. Allen is a prolific scholar whose current research falls under the rubric of "correctional mental health" and is directed at improving the lives of people with mental illness and those confined to mental health control units. His teaching includes a variety of courses, and he supervises a range of doctoral students nationally and internationally.

Em Olivia Bevis, EdD, RN, FAAN, had a lengthy and influential career in nursing education. An admired teacher and consultant, she spoke frequently on the need to infuse new pedagogies into nursing curricula and to cultivate caring communities among students and teachers. She authored several classic books and articles, including three editions of *Curriculum Building in Nursing: A Process*; "All in All It Was a Pretty Good Funeral" (*Journal of Nursing Education, 32*(3), 1993, pp. 99-100), and *Toward a Caring Curriculum: A New Pedagogy for Nursing* (coauthored with Jean Watson), which was awarded the 1990 *American Journal of Nursing* Book of the Year award. She was the recipient of numerous awards in recognition of her excellence in teaching, leadership, and service.

Peggy L. Chinn, PhD, RN, FAAN, is professor emerita of nursing at the University of Connecticut. Her BS in nursing is from the University of Hawaii, and master's and PhD degrees from the University of Utah. She authors books and journal articles on nursing theory, feminism and nursing, the art of nursing, and nursing education. Her major books, *Integrated Theory and Knowledge Development in Nursing* (7th ed., 2007), and *Peace and Power: Creative Leadership for Building Communities* (6th ed., 2007), are used worldwide. Her current focus for activism is the Nurse Manifest Project, a web-based project (www. nursemanifest.com) to inspire grassroots action by nurses to shape the future of nursing and health care. Cofounded with Richard Cowling (Virginia Commonwealth University) and Sue Hagedorn (University of Colorado), the project incorporates *Peace and Power* approaches to creating change. Dr. Chinn plays the harp, quilts, drums, and is an avid fan of women's music.

Nancy L. Diekelmann, PhD, RN, FAAN, is Helen Denne Schulte Professor Emerita at the University of Wisconsin-Madison School of Nursing and a fellow in the American Academy of Nursing, past president of the Society for Research in Nursing Education, and chair of the University of Wisconsin-Madison Teaching Academy. A noted authority for her work in nursing education and primary health care, Dr. Diekelmann has received two Book of the Year awards from the *American Journal of Nursing* for her textbooks *Primary Health Care of the Well Adult* and *Transforming RN Education: Dialogue and Debate* (coauthored with Marsha L. Rather). She received the National League for Nursing Excellence in Nursing Education Research award in 2001. Dr. Diekelmann was awarded the Doctor of Humane Letters in 2007 by the State University of New York at Farmingdale. Her current research uses hermeneutic phenomenology to explicate the narrative of students, teachers, and clinicians in nursing education toward a science of nursing education. Dr. Diekelmann has developed a research-based new pedagogy for nursing education: Narrative Pedagogy. She is co-author with John Diekelmann of a forthcoming book – *Schooling Learning Teaching: Toward Narrative Pedagogy.*

Jennie Gunn, PhD, CFNP, is an assistant professor of nursing at the University of Mississippi in Oxford. Dr. Gunn received her baccalaureate degree in nursing from the University of Southern Mississippi, graduating with highest honors. She earned her master's degree and PhD in nursing from the University of Mississippi Medical Center. She has authored many journal and newspaper articles, several southern cultural plays, and a book. Her major interests include educational and cultural research. Her hobbies include playing the violin and writing both fiction and nonfiction. Dr. Gunn received the Rene Reeb Award for Qualitative Research in 2005 and 2006.

Pamela M. Ironside, PhD, RN, FAAN, is an associate professor and director of the Center for Research in Nursing Education at the Indiana University School of Nursing. A consistent advocate for advancing an inclusive science of nursing education, Dr. Ironside is at the forefront of a national effort to bring research-based, discipline-specific pedagogies into nursing curricula and respond to challenges from contemporary practice environments. Her research with pilot schools worldwide that are enacting Narrative Pedagogy documents the contributions of reform using interpretive pedagogies and how it influences students' thinking. Her research substantively contributes to evidence-based approaches to faculty development in order to increase pedagogical literacy in nursing faculty. Her studies reflect research-based, multi-pedagogical practical strategies for all types of nursing programs that prepare students to practice amidst the uncertainty and ambiguity of the changing health care system. This research has been widely disseminated nationally and internationally via publications, lectures, workshops, and institutes.

Beverly Malone, PhD, RN, FAAN, began her nursing career with a first degree in nursing from the University of Cincinnati in 1970. She combined further study with clinical practice, a master's in psychiatric nursing, and received her doctorate in clinical psychology in 1981. Her career has mixed policy, education, administration, and clinical practice. Dr. Malone has worked as a surgical staff nurse, clinical nurse specialist, director of nursing, and assistant administrator of nursing. During the 1980s, she was dean of the School of Nursing at North Carolina Agricultural and Technical State University. In 1996, she was elected for two terms as president of the American Nurses Association (ANA), representing 180,000 nurses in the USA. In 2000, she became deputy assistant secretary for health within the US Department of Health and Human Services, the highest position so far held by any nurse in the US government. Dr. Malone was general secretary of the Royal College of Nursing (RCN), the United Kingdom's largest professional union of nurses, with more than 390,000 members, from June 2001 until January 2007. Dr Malone was also a member of the Higher Education Funding Council for England (HEFCE). She represented the RCN at the pan-European nursing body, the European Federation of Nurses Associations (EFN), the Commonwealth Nurses Federation, and the International Council of Nurses with the RCN president. In February 2007, Dr. Malone took up her appointment as chief executive officer of the National League for Nursing in New York.

Jane Sumner, PhD, RN, APRN, BC, is a professor and acting associate dean for undergraduate programs at the Louisiana State University Health Science Center School of Nursing in New Orleans. Her scholarship is in caring in nursing, her theory has been published, and she is pilot testing an instrument she developed to test her theory. Dr. Sumner utilizes critical social theory as a method to investigate issues in nursing and nursing education. Her education model, Quadrangular Dialogue, is in use in several US schools of nursing. She has presented her work many times internationally. Dr Sumner has specialist certification in community health nursing, and she is course coordinator for the master's program of public health/community health nursing Louisiana State. Most of her undergraduate teaching has been in the fundamentals of nursing; she does doctoral teaching as well. Dr. Sumner has served as chair of the NLN's Nurse Educator Workforce Development Advisory Council, and she is currently a member of the NLN Board of Governors.

M. Elaine Tagliareni, EdD, RN, is currently a Professor of Nursing and the Independence Foundation Chair in Community Health Nursing Education at Community College of Philadelphia. Dr. Tagliareni has been an associate degree nursing educator for more than 25 years. She received her BSN from Georgetown University School of Nursing, a master's degree in Mental Health and Community Nursing from the University of California, San Francisco and her doctorate from Teachers College, Columbia University with an emphasis on the role of the nurse educator in community colleges. In 1998, she was awarded the National League for Nursing Mildred Montag Excellence in Leadership Award. Dr. Tagliareni has wide-ranging participation in the National League for Nursing, serving on the Council of Associate Degree Programs, the Nursing Education Advisory Council and as President-elect. She will serve as President of the NLN in 2007-2009. She has played a key role in fostering innovation in nursing education and in promoting the nurse educator role as an advanced practice role. As President, Dr. Tagliareni will continue to advocate for excellence in nursing education through pedagogical research and to promote dialogue about successful strategies to prepare a diverse nursing workforce.

Christine A. Tanner, PhD, RN, FAAN, is the Youmans-Spaulding Distinguished Professor at Oregon Health & Science University School of Nursing and directs the postmaster's certificate program in nursing education. She served in a variety of roles at OHSU including director of the Office of Research Development and associate dean for the Statewide Undergraduate Program, and is currently one of the leaders in the development of the innovative Oregon Consortium for Nursing Education. She was the author of the 2001 study *Oregon s Nursing Shortage: A Public Health Crisis in the Making*. Dr. Tanner has served as the senior editor of the *Journal of Nursing Education* since 1991. She has conducted research for more than 25 years on clinical judgment in nursing, culminating in numerous journal publications and four books, including the award-winning *Expertise in Nursing Practice: Caring, Clinical Judgment and Ethics*, coauthored with Patricia Benner and Kit Chesla. She is the 2005 recipient of the National League for Nursing Excellence in Nursing Education Research Award, and has consulted nationally and internationally with schools of nursing on clinical judgment, nursing education research, and curriculum development. Dr. Tanner is the mother of two teenagers, neither of whom has shown any interest in being a nurse!! She is also an avid skier and student of piano.

Theresa M. "Terry" Valiga, EdD, RN, FAAN, is the chief program officer at the National League for Nursing, where she has responsibility for the organization's professional development initiatives, certification program, pedagogical research projects, Academy of Nursing Education, Centers of Excellence program, and other education-focused initiatives. Prior to this appointment, Dr. Valiga held teaching and administrative positions in five different universities and, over the course of her 26-year teaching career, taught in baccalaureate and master's programs, served on doctoral dissertation committees, earned the rank of professor, and served in the roles of undergraduate and graduate program director, as well as dean. She has published widely on nursing education issues and cognitive/intellectual development, and the third edition of her co-authored book, *The New Leadership Challenge: Creating the Future of Nursing,* will be published in 2008. In addition, she has completed several research studies, presented at national and international conferences, served as a consultant to schools of nursing in and outside the United States, and received numerous awards, including the NLN's Isabel Stewart Award for Excellence in Education and Sigma Theta Tau's Elizabeth Russell Belford (Founders) Award for Excellence in Nursing Education.

Verle Waters, MS, RN, is dean emerita at Ohlone College in California. Her BS is from the University of Minnesota and her MA is from Columbia University, Teachers College. She is the recipient of the Mary Adelaide Nutting Award for outstanding leadership in nursing education and the Mildred Montag Excellence in Leadership Award for outstanding contributions to associate degree nursing. Throughout her career, she was active in the National League for Nursing, serving in a variety of capacities from the Board of Governors to chair of the Council for Associate Degree Programs. In her retirement, she continues to be active in the National League for Nursing by serving on the Centers of Excellence Program review panel.